INTEGRATED PHARMACEUTICAL MEDICINE SERIES: VOLUME 1

A Concise Guide to
Clinical Trials

J. Rick Turner PhD

ISBN: 0615507670
ISBN 13: 9780615507675

Table of Contents

Preface

BIOPHARMACEUTICAL DRUGS IMPROVE the health and well-being of people across the globe on a scale that is unrivaled by any other medical intervention. Before these drugs can be prescribed for patients by their doctors, they have to be approved for marketing by the respective country's regulatory agency. To gain marketing approval, they must go through an extremely rigorous process that investigates their safety and efficacy: This is the process of New Drug Development. The last stage of this long, complex, and expensive process involves conducting clinical trials, the topic of this book.

Successfully conducting clinical trials requires the interdisciplinary collaboration of individuals from many clinical and scientific disciplines and areas of operational expertise. These include medicine, information technology, ethics and law, statistics, clinical trial operations, data collection and management, regulatory science, and medical writing, to name just a few. Central aspects of conducting clinical trials are discussed in the following chapters, with the goals of making specialists from each of these areas aware of the contributions of their colleagues, and helping readers to appreciate that everyone involved in clinical research is working side-by-side toward a common goal--- improving the health, well-being, and longevity of millions of patients around the globe.

Thanks are expressed to Jim Kendall, Jason Parker, and Rich Thomas for their enthusiastic support of this project.

This is the first volume in a new series entitled "Integrated Pharmaceutical Medicine." Other volumes will follow at regular intervals.

Dedicated to Karen, Misty, Mishadow, Charlie, and Mac

Biopharmaceutical Clinical Trials

1.1 Introduction

CONDUCTING CLINICAL TRIALS is an interdisciplinary and collaborative endeavor. It requires skilled individuals from many fields, including medicine, information technology, ethics and law, statistics, clinical trial operations, data collection and management, regulatory science, and medical writing. Because of this complexity, in addition to the specific skills needed to perform a particular role, it is helpful to have a fundamental knowledge of other aspects of clinical trials. This will help you to appreciate that, whatever your role, you are working side-by-side with many colleagues to contribute to the health, well-being, and longevity of millions of patients around the globe.

It is appropriate to remind ourselves frequently that, while drug development is a long, expensive, and difficult undertaking, it makes an enormous difference to the health of people worldwide. It is a noble pursuit, and it is a privilege to be a part of this process. However, with this privilege comes the responsibility to conduct our tasks to the highest ethical standards. Derenzo and Moss (2006) captured the importance of ethical considerations in all aspects of clinical studies:

> Each study component has an ethical aspect. The ethical aspects of a clinical trial cannot be separated from the scientific objectives. Segregation of ethical issues from the full range of study design components demonstrates a flaw in understanding the fundamental nature of research involving human subjects. Compartmentalization of ethical issues is inconsistent with a well-run trial. Ethical and scientific considerations are intertwined (p. 4).

1.2 Notes on Nomenclature

Several widely used terms are introduced in this section and defined as used in this book.

1.2.1 Drug

The term drug is used in this book to refer to traditional small-molecule drugs and also to biologics. Not surprisingly given their name, small-molecule drugs have a small molecular size and a low molecular weight. A typical definition would be molecules with a molecular weight less than 700 daltons (Da). While various definitions of a biologic can be found in the literature, it generally refers to medicinal products derived from blood, as well as vaccines and allergen products. Biologics tend to have considerably higher molecular weights. For example, monoclonal antibodies can have molecular weights in excess of 140,000 Da. While there are some important differences between these two categories of drugs, the clinical trial process is similar for both of them, and the discussions in this book pertain equally well to both.

1.2.2 Clinical Trial

Piantadosi (2005) provided a useful and succinct definition of a clinical trial: "A clinical trial is an experiment testing a medical treatment on human subjects (p. 16)." The term experiment conveys a study in which the researchers prospectively control the influence of interest. In the clinical trials of central interest in this book, certain subjects will be administered the new drug, while others will be administered a placebo, a matching tablet that has no pharmacological action. This straightforward study design allows the presentation of fundamental concepts that readily transfer to other equally important but somewhat more complex designs. At the end of such a trial the biological responses of subjects who were administered the drug will be compared with those of the subjects administered the placebo to see if the drug systematically exerted an influence on responses (e.g., lowered blood pressure, lessened pain, increased high-density lipoprotein cholesterol, or HDLc, the 'good cholesterol').

The term medical treatment addresses the fact that experiments can be conducted for other types of medical treatments, e.g., medical devices. The word human is used to distinguish clinical research from nonclinical research (sometimes called preclinical research) involving animals. Nonclinical research can evoke strong emotions, but it is the case that, at the present time, regulatory agencies (governmental agencies that provide oversight of drug development and ultimately decide if a new drug can be marketed) require that nonclinical research is performed before the drug can be administered to humans in clinical trials.

The word subject conveys that anyone taking part in clinical trials is, at that point in time, an experimental subject. Even if the person is under the care of a personal physician at the time of being recruited to take part in the trial, and is therefore a patient in that context, while participating in the trial the term subject is appropriate, even if it sounds a little impersonal. Clinical trials are experiments, and those taking part are experimental subjects.

1.2.3 Safety and Efficacy

Clinical trials examine the safety and efficacy of drugs in human subjects. Preapproval trials are conducted before the drug is approved by a regulatory agency for marketing. Postmarketing trials are conducted once the drug has been marketed and is being prescribed by physicians and taken by patients. Postmarketing trials, along with postmarketing surveillance, reflect the fact that drug development is a lifecycle process, not a process that stops at the time of marketing approval. It is important to continue to monitor safety and efficacy as long as the drug is on the market. As noted by the Institute of Medicine (IOM), "The approval decision does not represent a singular moment of clarity about the risks and benefits associated with a drug—preapproval clinical trials do not obviate continuing formal evaluation after approval" (IOM, 2007).

The term efficacy refers to a drug's ability to do what it is intended to do. For example, a drug for high blood pressure (hypertension) needs to lower blood pressure to demonstrate efficacy. The more blood pressure is lowered, the greater the degree of efficacy. In other words, efficacy is a measure of the drug's beneficial therapeutic action with regard to the disease or condition of clinical concern for which the drug is being developed. More succinctly, it is a measure of benefit.

While a drug's efficacy is important, its safety is more so. However, the definition of safety is not as straightforward as that for efficacy. It must be acknowledged that no drug is immune from the possibility of causing adverse reactions in certain individuals who are genetically and/or environmentally susceptible. One relatively simple but nonetheless meaningful conceptualization of safety is as the inverse of harm: the less harm a drug causes, the greater its safety: what is actually measured and recorded during clinical trials can be better described as drug harm. However, in practical terms, two considerations that would argue against this term come quickly to mind. First, it may seem strange to some to define something (safety) in terms of the absence of something else (harm). Second, while drug safety has legitimately attracted considerable attention among many stakeholders, it has accordingly become a high profile topic in many mass communication media. In this context, the term drug harm would likely be incendiary, attracting even more emotive behavior and sensationalism to an area already fueled by far too much of both. The assessment, discussion, and communication of drug safety issues must be approached in a calm, scientific manner.

A useful definition of drug safety was provided in the FDA's Sentinel Initiative (2008):

> Although marketed medical products are required by federal law to be safe for their intended use, **safety**

does not mean zero risk. A safe product is one that has acceptable risks, given the magnitude of benefit expected in a specific population and within the context of alternatives available.

Evaluation of drug safety and efficacy is discussed in more detail in Chapters 6 and 7. Part of the integrative discussion in Chapter 8 then focuses on the concept of benefit-risk assessment. We noted just a few moments ago that efficacy is a measure of benefit, and efficacy is therefore one of the components in assessment of benefit-risk balance. The risk component is related to drug safety: the more harm that is associated with the drug, the greater the risk it poses.

While the term "acceptable risk" in the quote from the Sentinel Initiative may at first seem strange, as we have already noted it is not possible to guarantee that a drug carries no risk to anyone. However, the benefits of a drug may far outweigh any risks, leading to the drug being approved. This decision is made at the public health level: the 'greater good is served' since many more people will receive benefit than will be harmed. If this seems in any way callous, consider how many individuals are killed in automobile accidents a year. Motorized transport is considered to serve the greater good, since many more people receive benefit from them (e.g., traveling to work to earn a living, visiting loved ones who are in hospital) than are harmed by them.

A different version of the same process of balancing likely benefits and possible risks occurs when a physician and patient decide together whether or not the patient should embark on a particular course of pharmacotherapy. In their considered opinion, the likely benefits must outweigh the possible risks. Just how much the benefits should outweigh the risks is determined on a case-by-case basis, and other factors such as the severity of the disease in question and the availability of other treatment options are part of each decision.

1.2.4 Contract Research Organization and Sponsor

A contract research organization (CRO) is a specialist company that conducts clinical research for drug companies (note that the C in the acronym stands for contract and not clinical). In this context, the term sponsor is used to refer to a drug company that has contracted a CRO to conduct clinical research, such as a clinical trial.

The traditional model by which sponsors and CROs worked together is one in which CROs were hired by sponsors as service providers, providing a prespecified set of services exactly as requested for a given fee. A more recent model is one in which the CRO functions as a full drug development partner. In this latter model a sponsor and its CRO start working together, ideally as soon as the sponsor conceptualizes a clinical trial. While the sponsor may have expertise in many aspects of study design and operational execution 'in house,' a good CRO will also have expertise in all of these aspects and can therefore provide additional (and sometimes unique) beneficial input into the planning of the trial.

1.2.5 The Study Protocol

The Study Protocol is "the most important document in clinical trials, since it ensures the quality and integrity of the clinical investigation in terms of its planning, execution, conduct, and the analysis of the data" (Chow and Chang, 2007). The study protocol is a comprehensive plan of action that contains information concerning the goals of the study, details of subject recruitment, details of safety monitoring, and all aspects of design, methodology, and analysis. (In some cases, a Statistical Analysis Plan, associated with and written at the same time as the study protocol, will contain the detailed description of the analyses to be conducted.) Input is therefore required, for example, from clinical scientists, medical safety officers, study managers, data managers, and statisticians. Consequently, while one clinical scientist or medical writer may take primary responsibility for the protocol's preparation, many members of the study team make important contributions.

The requirements of a study protocol include:

- Objectives (usually Primary and Secondary objectives). These goals of the study are stated as precisely as possible.
- Measurements related to the drug's safety, and procedures to ensure the safety of all subjects while participating in the trial.
- Inclusion and exclusion criteria. These provide detailed criteria for subject eligibility for participation in the trial.
- Details of the procedures for physical examinations.
- Laboratory procedures. Full details of the nature and timing of all procedures and tests are provided.
- Electrocardiogram (ECG) measurement, and any other measurements such as imaging.
- Drug treatment schedule. Route of administration, dosage, and dosing regimen are detailed. This information is also provided for the control treatment.
- In the case of later-phase trials, measurements of efficacy (the different phases are described shortly in Section 1.4). The criteria to be used to determine efficacy are provided.
- In the case of later-phase trials, details of the method of diagnosis of the disease or condition of clinical concern for which the drug is intended.
- Statistical analysis. The precise analytical strategy needs to be detailed, here and/or in an associated statistical analysis plan.

Inclusion and exclusion criteria are central components of clinical trials. A study's inclusion and exclusion criteria govern which individuals interested in participating in the trial are admitted to the study as subjects. Criteria for inclusion in the study include items such as the following:

- Reliable evidence of a diagnosis of the disease or condition of clinical concern.
- Being within the specified age range.

- Willingness to take measures to prevent pregnancy during the course of treatment. This includes a female in the trial not becoming pregnant (she may be receiving the drug being tested), and a male participating in the trial not causing a female to become pregnant (he may be receiving the drug being tested).

Criteria for exclusion from the study include:

- Taking certain medications for other medical conditions and which therefore cannot safely be stopped during the trial.
- Participation in another clinical trial within so many months prior to the commencement of this study.
- Liver or kidney disease.

While inclusion and exclusion criteria are typically provided in two separate lists in regulatory documentation, exclusion criteria can be regarded as further refinements of the inclusion criteria. Meeting all the inclusion criteria allows a subject to be considered as a study participant, while not meeting any exclusion criteria is also necessary to allow the subject to become a participant.

1.3 General Anatomy of a Clinical Trial

The anatomy of a clinical trial can be represented by a model comprising three components:

- Study design: It is critical to use a design that will facilitate the collection of required data.
- Trial conduct: This comprises employing optimum quality experimental methodology and optimum quality operational execution. The former means that optimum quality data **can** be collected, and the latter ensures that such data **are indeed** collected.
- Analysis of the data collected and interpretation of these analyses in the context of the research question the trial has been designed to answer.

While different types of clinical trials have different goals (as discussed in the next section) they all have several characteristics in common, including:

- A research question. There must always be a defined purpose for conducting, or running, a clinical trial, and this is captured by the research question.
- A study design. The trial has to be designed so that it will facilitate the collection of optimum quality data with which to answer the research question being asked.
- Trial execution (running the trial). This requires optimum quality experimental methodology (e.g., employment of equipment that has been validated to measure blood pressure accurately when used correctly) and first-rate operational execution (e.g., actually using the blood pressure measuring equipment correctly, getting the test drug to all of the hospitals, academic research centers, and physicians' offices where the trial is being run on schedule, and a multitude of other tasks).
- Data storage and management.
- Statistical analysis of the data collected, and skillful interpretation of these numerical results to provide the most informative and clinically meaningful answer to the research question.

These components operate together in a process that is integrative, interactive, and, ideally, seamless. Study design, experimental methodology, operational execution, and statistical analysis and interpretation are central characters in the development of new drugs, all playing their roles in the collection of optimum quality data with which to answer research questions of interest during the drug's clinical development program.

At this point, allow me to interject a request: Please don't start worrying because you have just seen the word 'statistics' in the previous list of bullet points. You may have taken some courses in this subject and then decided that statistics is definitely something for 'someone else' to worry about! Please allow me approach the subject from a different perspective. The discipline of Statistics (deliberately written with an upper-case S to denote that it is a scientific discipline in its own right, not just a set of rules by which to calculate some results given a bunch of data) provides an excellent way to make rational, informed decisions, and such decisions are needed throughout drug development. It is also a central component of clinical trials, and professional statisticians need to be involved from the start all the way to writing reports of the trial and its results and interpretation. Having said that, in this book only a couple of basic statistical concepts will be discussed, and, in addition to an appreciation of and respect for its central importance, that will be all that most of you need to know about Statistics.

1.4 Clinical Trial Phases

Many different clinical trials are conducted to examine the safety and efficacy of a drug. (The term investigational drug is often used in this context to denote a drug that has moved into clinical trials following the successful completion of its nonclinical development program.) Among the goals of a drug's clinical development program are the following:

- Estimation of the investigational drug's safety and tolerance in healthy adults.
- Determination of a safe and effective dose range, safe dosing levels, and the preferred route of administration.
- Investigation of pharmacokinetics and pharmacodynamics following a single-dose and a multiple-dose schedule.
- Establishment and validation of biochemical markers in body fluids that may permit the assessment of the drug's desired pharmacological activity.
- Identification of metabolic pathways relevant to the drug.
- Continued evaluation of the drug's safety and an initial evaluation of efficacy in a relatively small group of subjects with the

disease or condition of clinical concern (the targeted therapeutic indication).

- Selection and optimization of final formulations, doses, regimens, and efficacy endpoints for larger scale, multicenter studies. Efficacy endpoints should be able to be measured reliably and should quantitatively reflect clinically relevant changes in the disease or condition of clinical concern.
- Evaluation of the drug's comparative efficacy (measured against placebo or an active comparator, i.e., a drug that is already on the market) in larger scale, multicenter studies, and collection of additional safety data.

Clinical trials are often categorized into four phases, Phases I–IV. (Sometimes additional sub-categorization is provided by adding an "a" or a "b" to one of these.) Typical descriptions of these phases are:

- Phase I: Pharmacologically oriented studies that typically look for the best dose to employ. Comparison with other treatments is not typically built into the study design.
- Phase II: Trials that look for evidence of biological activity, efficacy, and safety at a fixed dose. Again, comparison with other treatments is not typically built into the study design.
- Phase III: Trials in which comparison with another treatment (e.g., a placebo) is a fundamental component of the design. These trials are undertaken if Phase I and Phase II studies have provided preliminary evidence that the investigational drug is safe and effective.
- Phase IV: These are postmarketing trials, conducted after the drug has been approved to collect additional information about drug responses in groups of individuals who may have been excluded from preapproval trials.

Another categorization system has been suggested by an organization with a long name but a thankfully short abbreviation—the International

Conference on Harmonisation of Technical Requirements for Registration of Pharmaceuticals for Human Use (ICH). This collaboration comprises regulatory agencies and industry organizations from the United States, Europe, and Japan (historically the largest pharmaceutical markets). ICH's goal is to make regulatory processes more similar across the board, and hence to reduce or obviate the need to duplicate the animal and human testing carried out during drug development. Their categorization system is shown in Table 1.1. The four categories correspond closely to Phases I-IV as just described, but in this case their titles convey meaningful information about the trials in the respective categories.

Table 1.1: Classifying Clinical Studies According to Their Objectives

Objective of Trials	Study Examples
Human Pharmacology • Assess tolerance. • Describe or define pharmacokinetics (PK) and pharmacodynamics (PD). • Explore drug metabolism and drug interactions. • Estimate (biological) activity.	• Dose-tolerance studies. • Single- and multiple-dose PK and/or PD studies. • Drug interaction studies.
Therapeutic Exploratory • Explore use for the targeted indication. • Estimate dosage for subsequent studies. • Provide basis for confirmatory study design, endpoints, methodologies.	• Earliest trials of relatively short duration in well-defined narrow populations with the disease or condition of clinical concern, using surrogate of pharmacological endpoints or clinical measures. • Dose-response exploration studies.

Objective of Trials	Study Examples
Therapeutic Confirmatory • Demonstrate/confirm efficacy. • Establish safety profile. • Provide an adequate basis for assessing benefit/risk relationship to support licensing (market approval). • Establish dose-response relationship.	• Adequate and well-controlled studies to establish efficacy. • Randomized parallel dose-response studies. • Clinical safety studies. • Studies of mortality/morbidity outcomes. • Large simple trials. • Comparative studies
Therapeutic Use • Refine understanding of benefit-risk relationship in general or special populations and/or environments. • Identify less common adverse drug reactions. • Refine dosing recommendations.	• Comparative effectiveness studies • Studies of mortality/morbidity outcomes • Studies of additional endpoints. • Large simple trials. • Pharmaco-economic studies.

Based on ICH E8: General Considerations for Clinical Trials. See www.ich.org

1.4.1 Human Pharmacology (Phase I) Trials

Initial safety evaluations are conducted in healthy adult subjects in first-time-in-human studies, abbreviated as FTIH studies or often just FIH studies. The term 'normal volunteers' is often used for the individuals participating in these trials, but (at least to this author) it is misleading and somewhat disrespectful. The process of enrolling subjects into clinical trials (subject recruitment) requires that subjects be treated with the upmost respect: without their voluntary participation clinical trials cannot be conducted. A key concept is informed consent, which is operationalized by subjects reading a document describing the nature and requirements of the trial, asking questions and receiving answers to their satisfaction, and acknowledging (via signature of an Informed Consent Form) that they have been so informed and are participating voluntarily. By definition, therefore, all subjects in all clinical trials are volunteers (a central component of ethically conducted trials), and the use of the term volunteer only in the context of FIH trials could be taken to imply that participants in other trials are not volunteers. Additionally, the term normal could be taken to imply that subjects in other trials are abnormal in ways not related to having or not having the disease or condition of clinical concern. The term healthy adult subjects, therefore, has considerable merit.

Human pharmacology (Phase I) studies assess the safety of the drug, obtain a thorough knowledge and understanding of the drug's pharmacokinetic profile (absorption, distribution, metabolism, and excretion) and potential interactions with other drugs, and estimate pharmacodynamic activity, i.e., drug-induced biological activity. They are typically conducted by clinical pharmacologists. A range of doses and/or dosing intervals is investigated in a sequential manner. Characterization of the drug's safety profile may include investigation of pharmacokinetics, structure-activity relationships, mechanisms of action, and identifying preferred routes of administration and potential interactions with other medications.

Typically, between 20 and 80 healthy adults (this number can certainly be lower) participate in these relatively short studies, and subjects are often recruited from university medical school settings where trials are being conducted. Subjects are given extensive physical examinations before and after administration of the drug and, in the case of longer term studies, at various intervals throughout the treatment. An extensive battery of typical tests includes:

- Liver function.
- Kidney function.
- Blood chemistry.
- Urine chemistry.
- Eye testing.
- ECG readings.
- Others specific to target organ systems.

Acute single-dose studies are conducted first, with the dose used based on extrapolation from the nonclinical studies that preceded the commencement of FIH studies (while certainly not perfect, this extrapolation provides the best information for this purpose that is available at the time). Short-term studies of various doses follow, and then longer-term studies of various doses are conducted. Eventually, dose-finding studies are conducted to determine the maximum tolerated dose (MTD) of the drug. These studies facilitate the examination of pharmacokinetic parameters and toxicity. They are informative with regard to providing answers to questions concerning the side effects that are seen, their characteristics, and whether they are consistent to any notable degree across subjects.

As alluded to previously, no animal model is a perfect predictor of the precise effects of the drug in humans, and there is always the possibility that serious safety issues may arise during human pharmacology trials. For example, a trial involving an investigational drug known as TGN1412 was conducted in March 2006. Subjects administered the drug experienced rapidly developing, extremely serious adverse events, some of which had long-term consequences for subjects' health (Nada and Somberg, 2007). Fortunately, such occurrences are very rare.

1.4.2 Therapeutic Exploratory (Phase II) Trials

Therapeutic exploratory studies examining efficacy (and continuing to add information to the accumulating safety profile) are typically conducted by individuals specifically trained in clinical trial methodology and execution. Some authors have voiced the opinion that these trials provide the most accurate assessment of efficacy, since they are conducted in an extremely tightly controlled manner (other authors have noted that, while this is likely true, this environment is not typical of those in which the drug will eventually be used if approved).

Several hundred subjects with the disease or clinical condition for which the drug is being developed participate in these trials, along with a similar number of subjects who receive a different drug, the control treatment (e.g., a placebo) against which the drug being developed is compared. This comparator, also known as the control treatment, can be a placebo, a compound with no pharmacological activity, or an active control, i.e., a different drug that has a known pharmacological activity.

1.4.3 Therapeutic Confirmatory (Phase III) Trials

Therapeutic confirmatory studies are typically run as double-blind, randomized, concurrently controlled clinical trials once human pharmacology and therapeutic exploratory studies have defined the most likely safe and effective dosage regimens to be used (these terms are all explained in due course). Several thousand subjects with the disease or clinical condition for which the drug is being developed participate, along with a similar number of subjects who receive a control treatment. Additional safety data are gained from these trials, adding to the accumulating safety data portfolio.

The technique of randomization places subjects who are recruited into a clinical trial into one of the treatment groups at random. As an extreme example, if there are two treatment groups in a trial we do not want all males in one treatment group and all females in the other treatment group: any result obtained could be heavily influenced by this disparity between groups. Randomization is therefore employed to ensure that the members of the groups are as similar as possible with one exception, i.e., the treatment they receive during the trial. It is generally acknowledged that the first randomized clinical trial, conducted in the late 1940s, was a study evaluating the use of streptomycin in treating tuberculosis conducted by the (British) Medical Research Council Streptomycin in Tuberculosis Trials Committee.

While trials conducted in all phases are important, discussion of all phases are not possible in a book of this length. Discussions therefore focus on Phase III trials.

1.4.4. Therapeutic Use (Phase IV) Trials

Therapeutic use studies are conducted once the drug is on the market. They may be optional studies conducted by the sponsor, or studies required by a regulatory agency as a condition of approving the drug for marketing. In the former case the sponsor may wish to know more about the drug's performance in patients who were not well represented in the Phase III trials, e.g., an older population if the exclusion criteria excluded people of the age now of interest, patients with compromised liver function, and patients taking one or more concomitant medications. In the latter, the regulatory agency approving the drug for marketing felt that, based upon the benefit-risk balance of the drug as indicated by the data they had to review at that time, the drug could be marketed and hence offer benefit to patients, but also felt that it would be advantageous to require the sponsor to provide additional information.

1.5 Ethical Considerations

Before concluding this introductory chapter, the paramount need for the highest ethical standards in designing, executing, analyzing, and reporting the results of clinical trials must be emphasized. This topic was raised at the start of this chapter in Section 1.1, and will be addressed again in the final chapter. Every aspect of clinical trials has ethical demands, and you will become conversant with these as you learn more about clinical research. The often-cited fundamental ethical principles include equipoise, respect for persons, beneficence, and justice. However, there are a multitude of other instances that require ethical conduct. For example, when designing a trial, its design must be capable of producing optimum quality biological information (data) that allow the research question to be answered in an optimum way. If, despite flawless research methodology and operational execution, the data acquired do not permit the research question asked to be answered in an appropriate manner, the expectations of the subjects who participated in the trial to advance medical knowledge have been violated, and they have been exposed to potential harm (side effects) unnecessarily and unethically.

CHAPTER 2

The Regulatory Environment

2.1 Introduction

THE RELEVANCE AND importance of the regulatory environment in which clinical trials are conducted cannot be overemphasized. It is largely a result of the ICH, which, as was noted in the previous chapter, is an amalgamation of expertise from various regulatory agencies and pharmaceutical organizations across the world.

The ICH arose since the regulations for submitting documentation requesting marketing approval of a drug were historically quite different between countries. Data requirements around the world were dissimilar, meaning that studies often had to be repeated to satisfy differing national regulatory requirements if marketing permission was desired in multiple countries. This lack of uniformity meant that bringing a drug to market in various countries took longer than necessary, delaying its availability to patients.

Harmonization of regulatory requirements was pioneered by the European Community (now the European Union) in the 1980s, as it moved towards the development of a single market for pharmaceuticals. The success achieved in Europe demonstrated that harmonization was feasible. The harmonization process was then extended to include Japan and the United States. The regulatory agencies in these three geographic regions are the European Medicines Agency, the Pharmaceuticals and Medical Devices Agency, and the Food and Drug Administration, respectively.

Sponsors and regulatory agencies each have roles and responsibilities for drug products. Marketing approval of a drug is a contract between the sponsor and the regulatory agency, and the conditions of the approval are spelled out in detail and also condensed in the prescribing information. Any planned changes on the part of the sponsor need to be presented to the agency, and new approval is necessary in many cases. A regulatory agency's roles and responsibilities include:

- Approving drugs that have been scientifically evaluated to provide evidence of a satisfactory benefit-risk ratio (the balance between the therapeutic advantages of receiving the drug and possible risks).
- Monitoring the safety of the marketed drug. (Although it tends to receive less attention, lack of expected efficacy can also be regarded as a safety issue, since patients would not be receiving the expected benefit, leaving their disease essentially untreated.)
- In serious cases, withdrawing the license for marketing. This can occur for various reasons, including failure of adequate additional information being included in the prescribing information after adverse reactions are reported and failure to be compliant with regulations concerning drug manufacture.

A sponsor's roles and responsibilities include:

- Keeping all pertinent documentation related to the drug up to date and ensuring it complies with standards set by the current state of scientific knowledge and the regulatory agency.
- Collecting, compiling, and evaluating safety data and submitting regular reports to the regulatory agency.
- Taking rapid action where necessary. This includes withdrawal of a particular batch of the drug or withdrawal of the entire product if warranted.

2.1.1 Goals of the ICH

The ICH has several goals, including:

- Maintaining a forum for a constructive dialog between regulatory authorities and the pharmaceutical industry on differences in technical requirements for marketing approval in the

European Union, the United States, and Japan to ensure a more timely introduction of new drugs and hence their availability to patients.

- Facilitating the adoption of new or improved technical research and development (R&D) approaches that update or replace current practices. These new or improved practices should permit a more economical use of animal, human, and material resources without compromising safety.
- Monitoring and updating harmonized technical requirements leading to a greater mutual acceptance of R&D data.
- Contributing to the protection of public health from an international perspective.
- Encouraging the implementation and integration of common standards of documentation and submission of regulatory applications by disseminating harmonized guidelines.

To facilitate the last goal, the ICH has produced many guidance documents for sponsors to use in various aspects of drug development research and documentation, including drug safety, efficacy, and quality. Readers are referred to the ICH web site, www.ich.org, for more detailed information.

2.2 The US Food and Drug Administration

The regulatory agency responsible for the governance of new drug development in the United States is the Food and Drug Administration (FDA). Since the author works in the United States, this agency is the focus of discussions. However, the general principles of regulatory affairs and the regulatory landscapes in which clinical trials are conducted are relatively similar across various regulatory agencies.

The FDA's relatively broad mission includes providing reasonable assurances that drugs are safe and effective. Two program centers facilitate the FDA's involvement in biopharmaceutical development and use:

- The Center for Drug Evaluation and Research (CDER).
- The Center for Biologics Evaluation and Research (CBER).

The FDA also oversees drug manufacturing. While primarily (and correctly) regarded as a regulatory agency, the FDA is also a law enforcement agency. If its preferred administrative methods do not achieve satisfactory outcomes, it can utilize the US court system and the Department of Justice's assistance to invoke its judicial tools, which include seizure, injunction, and prosecution.

2.3 Regulatory Requirements, Documentation, and Pathway to Drug Approval

The FDA's new drug development and approval process includes several principal steps:

- A sponsor's submission of an Investigational New Drug Application (IND: note that there is no A at the end of this abbreviation) following the completion of nonclinical research.
- FDA review of the IND.
- Preparation and submission of a New Drug Application (NDA) for small-molecule drugs or a Biologics License Application (BLA) for biologics following clinical research.
- FDA review and approval of the NDA or BLA. Following an initial review, the agency may ask for more documentation before granting marketing approval.

There are many regulatory requirements for new drug development and approval. While processes must be conducted as required, their conduct and completion by itself is not sufficient: appropriate documentation is critical. From the regulatory perspective, if something that should be documented is not documented, for all intents and purposes it has not been done. Virtually everyone involved in conducting clinical trials is required to keep detailed records of their activities and actions.

2.3.1 The Investigational New Drug Application

Technically, an IND is a request for an exemption from a particular federal statute. Current federal law requires that a drug has to have been approved for marketing before it can be transported or distributed across state lines. Therefore, officially, a drug that is being tested in preapproval clinical trials cannot be shipped across state lines in interstate commerce because, by definition, it has not been approved for marketing. Most Phase II and Phase III trials are conducted in many states (and possibly many countries), and so sponsors will likely want to ship the investigational drug to clinical investigators in many states. The sponsor therefore has to request an exemption from the statute prohibiting this. The IND is the vehicle via which the sponsor technically obtains this exemption from the FDA.

In scientific terms, the purpose of an IND is to provide detailed documentation that will allow the FDA to conclude that it is reasonable for the sponsor to proceed to clinical trials. Generally, this includes data and information in four broad areas:

- Animal pharmacology and toxicology studies. These nonclinical data permit an assessment of whether the product is considered to be reasonably safe for initial testing in humans. The phrase 'considered to be reasonably safe' may sound somewhat less than definitive or reassuring, but it is simply the case that no amount of nonclinical testing can guarantee that a drug will be absolutely safe when administered to humans. As in many instances in the drug development process, an informed judgment has to be made, on this occasion by the regulatory agency.
- Manufacturing information. These data address the composition, manufacture, stability, and controls used for manufacturing the drug. This information is provided to document the sponsor's ability to produce and supply consistent batches of high-quality drug.

- Clinical study protocols. Protocols include precise accounts of the design, methodology, and analysis considerations necessary to conduct the proposed studies and analyze their results. Therefore, design, methodology, and analysis information must be submitted in study protocol format before administering the investigational drug to the first human subject. These detailed protocols for the proposed initial-phase clinical studies are provided to allow the FDA to assess whether the trials will expose subjects to unnecessary risks.
- Investigator information. Information on the qualifications of clinical investigators is provided to allow assessment of whether they are qualified to fulfill their duties at the investigational sites used during the clinical trials.

When submitting an IND, a sponsor should state the goals that make up the overall clinical development program. When originally submitted, the general investigational plan should outline the overall plan, but it only need articulate the studies to be conducted during the first year of clinical development. Subsequent IND updates provide additional details. The FDA's overall review process consists of several reviews, including medical/clinical, chemistry, pharmacology/toxicology, and statistical.

2.3.2 The New Drug Application

At the completion of a drug's clinical development program a New Drug Application (NDA: this time the acronym does include an "A") is filed. The regulations pertaining to NDAs provide detailed guidance for both content and format. Typically, sponsors meet with the FDA to discuss the content and format of an NDA prior to its preparation. Pre-NDA meetings can be crucial for the sponsor to understand the content and format that will best facilitate the review process for a given submission. The FDA's review of the NDA focuses on determining if it finds the evidence concerning safety, efficacy, and manufacturing ability to be compelling, and if it is therefore prepared to approve the drug for marketing.

Historically, NDAs, like other regulatory documents, were submitted on paper, and the total amount of paperwork was considerable. A typical paper NDA submission might constitute 400 volumes, each 400 pages long. The process has been moving toward electronic submission for some time, which has many advantages, including the fact that hyperlinks can be incorporated that allow a reviewer to navigate directly from one part of the submission to another. This is particularly valuable for statistical reviewers who may wish to navigate from the Methods section of a clinical study report (CSR) to tabulated data presented in the Results section and then to the supporting raw data sets.

CHAPTER 3

Study Design and
Experimental Methodology

3.1 Introduction

AS WAS SEEN in Chapter 1, many different kinds of clinical trials are conducted during a drug's clinical development program, with each being designed to answer a specific research question. This progression of trials facilitates incremental increases in knowledge about the safety and efficacy of the drug. Given this book's focus on Phase III trials, the discussions of study design and experimental methodology in this chapter are geared towards such trials. However, many general points are also applicable to trials in other phases.

3.2 The Randomized, Double-blind, Placebo-controlled, Parallel-groups Study

There are several kinds of study designs for Phase III trials, including superiority, equivalence, and non-inferiority designs. Historically, the superiority design was more commonly employed, but the other two designs are now increasingly used. Nonetheless, our discussions will focus on the superiority trial since the basic statistical principles of interest in this book can be introduced most simply in this context. Moreover, once you have a good understanding of these principles in the context of a superiority trial you will be able to readily translate your understanding of them with regard to equivalence and non-inferiority trials.

Superiority trials can take various forms. The study design frequently discussed in this book can be described by a collection of terms with which you will become familiar during the following chapters: the randomized, double-blind, controlled, parallel-groups study design. This design includes a drug treatment group in which subjects receive the drug and a separate group of subjects who receive a control drug. The control group discussed most frequently is a second group of subjects who receive a placebo. This group is referred to as the placebo treatment group. Other control groups can certainly be used, such as another drug for the same disease or condition of clinical concern. Since such a drug would be pharmacologically active, it is called an active control. Indeed, in certain settings it is unethical to use a placebo rather than an active control drug. One example is during the development of a drug for a serious disease such as cancer. In this setting the drug may be being developed as an 'add-on' treatment that will be added to the 'standard of care' or 'gold standard' treatment that is currently the treatment-of-choice for that particular cancer. Those in the drug treatment group will receive the standard of care treatment plus the new drug, while those in the other group (here called an active control group) will receive the standard of care therapy. Nonetheless, the points made in our discussions regarding the use of a placebo will provide a solid understanding of the comparative nature of Phase III trials.

3.2.1 Randomization and the Parallel-groups Design

Randomization is a process that facilitates the random and independent allocation of trial subjects to the different treatment groups in a parallel-group design before the commencement of the trial. In this study design, one group of subjects is randomized to the drug treatment group, hence being administered the drug during the trial, and a second group of subjects is randomized to the placebo treatment group, hence receiving the placebo during the trial. The influence of interest, the pharmacological effect of the drug under investigation, is therefore under the researchers' prospective control, since a certain identified group of subjects receive the drug treatment while another identified group of subjects receive the placebo treatment. If due attention is paid to methodological and statistical considerations, especially to randomization, differential physiological responses between these treatment groups can be attributed to the difference between the drug and the placebo.

3.2.2 Double-blind Strategy

Employing the double-blind methodology is a hallmark of Phase III trials. When responses to a drug are compared with responses to the placebo both drug products must be made to look, smell, and taste the same so that subjects cannot deduce from one of these characteristics which treatment they are receiving. These drug products must also be manufactured and shipped to the investigational sites used in the trial in a manner that does not allow the physician investigators to know which treatment each subject is being administered. Thus, both the subjects and those conducting the trial are 'blind' to which treatment the subjects are receiving.

3.2.3 Controlled Study

The term controlled study conveys that the drug is being compared against a control group. In our case, it is being compared against placebo. Going one step further, the term concurrently controlled study makes clear that the different groups take part in their respective treatment arms at the same time. If all of the subjects in one treatment group completed their participation first, and then all of the other subjects completed their participation at some later time it is quite possible that other factors could confound the results. On most occasions, however, the shorter term 'controlled study' is used, with the implicit expectation that all concerned will know that the two treatment groups participate concurrently.

3.3 Experimental Methodology

In the ideal conduct of a clinical trial, experimental methodology and operational execution combine together in a seamless fashion with a single goal, the acquisition of optimum quality data. In clinical trials the data acquired are numerical and descriptive representations of biologically and clinically important information. As noted in Section 1.3, acquiring optimum quality data in clinical trials requires two things. First, all measurement instruments must be capable of measuring parameters of interest accurately and reliably when used correctly. Second, first-rate operational execution must occur to make sure that these instruments are indeed used correctly on all occasions of measurement, and that all other operational requirements are executed flawlessly.

Experimental methodology's purpose is to exert as much control as possible over potentially confounding influences during the collection of the data. In more mathematical terms, it is to reduce variability in every possible influence with the exception of the influence of interest, i.e., the influence exerted by the drug. Analytical focus then falls on searching for any systematic variation in these data caused by the drug. To increase the chance of detecting any such systematic variation it is important to decrease to the greatest extent possible any random variation caused by all identifiable and controllable extraneous factors.

3.4 Variation in Data Sets

In any set of data, unless every value is precisely the same, there will be variation. Such variation can be captured by various statistics such as the range, variance, standard deviation, and standard error.

Imagine two sets of data representing blood pressure changes during a Phase III clinical trial for a new antihypertensive drug. The subjects in this trial will have the disease of concern, namely high blood pressure, also called hypertension. One set contains blood pressure change scores from the 1,500 subjects randomized into the drug treatment group, and the other contains similar data for the 1,500 subjects randomized into the placebo treatment group. They all received treatment (drug or placebo) for 12 weeks and their blood pressure at the end of the treatment period was compared with their baseline blood pressure, i.e., their blood pressure before the treatment started. Blood pressure assessment typically involves two values, systolic blood pressure (SBP) and diastolic blood pressure (DBP), both being measured in milliliters of mercury (mmHg). For ease of explanation of the statistical concepts being discussed here, the change in 'blood pressure' from the beginning to the end of the treatment period is considered as being represented by a single value for each subject. This is a legitimate strategy since the parameter called mean arterial pressure (MAP) is a single value computed from SBP and DBP.

Consider first the subjects in the drug treatment group. A change score for MAP was calculated for each subject as:

Change score = MAP at end-of-treatment minus MAP at baseline

For physiological reasons, the probability that all 1,500 subjects will show the same change in MAP is vanishingly small. Therefore, we will assume that there is variation in this dataset. The other dataset contains change scores in MAP for a separate group of 1,500 hypertensive individuals recruited into in the same clinical trial and randomized into the placebo treatment group. Even though these individuals received placebo treatment, it is likely that many (and possibly a majority) will have non-zero change scores, and it is again extremely unlikely that these changes will all be identical. Again, therefore, we will assume that there is variation in the data.

3.4.1 Systematic Influence and Random Error
The topic of statistical significance is addressed in Chapter 7 when discussing the provision of compelling evidence of efficacy. At this point, we will simply note that three factors are of central importance in determining the attainment of statistical significance:

1. Variation *between* the two sets of data, or between-groups variation;

2. Variation *within* the two sets of data, or within-groups variation;

3. The total number of subjects participating in the trial (the sum of subjects in each treatment group), sometimes expressed as the size of the trial.

The following statements can then be made for each of these factors, assuming in each case that the other two factors remain constant:

- The greater the between-groups variation (operationalized as the greater the difference between the group means, i.e., the greater the treatment effect), the **more** likely it is that the difference will attain statistical significance.

- The greater the within-groups variation, the **less** likely it is that the difference will attain statistical significance.

- The greater the number of subjects participating in the trial, the **more** likely it is that the difference will attain statistical significance.

Notice that two of these three factors address variation. Consider the first statement, which is intuitively the most straightforward. Using nomenclature introduced previously this statement can be reworded as follows: The larger the treatment effect, the more likely it is to attain statistical significance. That is, all other factors (including assessments of the drug's safety) being constant, the greater the drug's efficacy the more likely it is that regulators will consider the results to provide compelling evidence that the drug should receive marketing approval.

The influence of the drug, captured by the treatment effect, can be considered a systematic influence. It can also be regarded as the signal in which we are interested. In contrast, in the present context, the within-groups variation can be regarded as non-systematic variation, or the noise against which we desire to detect the signal. (The following section discusses this issue in a different context.) This noise has two components: biological variation and random error. Since we all have unique biological systems, including those pertinent to a drug's influence on the body (a statement that is true for identical twins and other identical births given the gene-environment interactions they experience), biological variation is inevitable and perfectly normal. It is the reason that Phase III trials typically contain several thousand subjects, since this many are required for the signal of interest to be detected against the noise.

In contrast, random error can be addressed. Indeed, *minimizing random error is the responsibility of each and every person involved in the planning and conduct of a clinical trial.* There are multiple instances where such error can occur, with the following being just a few examples:

- Administering the wrong drug treatment to a subject on one or more occasions during the trial.
- Employing measurement equipment that is sub-standard.
- Conducting blood pressure measurements in an inconsistent manner.
- Recording a measurement incorrectly.
- Misplacing data.
- Behaving in such a manner that one or more subjects decide for themselves (correctly or incorrectly) which treatment they are receiving.

The message here is simple: Optimum quality research methodology contributes to optimum quality data, and everyone must strive to the greatest extent possible to execute their role in the trial flawlessly to reduce random error, thus allowing the trial the best opportunity of accurately assessing the drug's characteristics.

3.5 Occasions When Within-group Variation is of Primary Interest

In the context of interest in the previous section it was noted that working diligently to minimize random error (with the goal of minimizing within-group variation) is important. In a different context, however, the within-group variation for the drug treatment group may be of specific interest. If it is reliably found in several trials that a drug demonstrates particularly strong efficacy in some individuals who can be identified prospectively while demonstrating considerably less efficacy in others, this finding is of interest in itself. (Identification may have been retrospective on the first occasion this differential response was suspected, but it must be found prospectively in subsequent trials for this observation to be meaningful.) For example, those who are likely to show particularly good responses to the drug may do so for genetic reasons that can be identified before commencing pharmacotherapy by a diagnostic test. This facilitates the practice of individualized medicine (other names seen in this context include personalized, stratified, and precision medicine).

CHAPTER 4

Operational Execution

4.1 Introduction

THE LOGISTICS OF operationally executing a clinical trial are enormous. Consider a Phase III trial involving 3,000 subjects participating at a total of 100 investigational sites that are spread across several continents. Identifying potential subjects and then recruiting and retaining the required number is one challenge. Shipping the drug products for the clinical trial to investigational sites located in various countries spread around the globe is another. Making sure that all necessary data are measured and recorded is a major task, as is managing and storing the data. And the list goes on. Of necessity, this chapter is far from exhaustive in its descriptions of operational aspects of running a clinical trial. Rather, its aim is to give you a feel for some the challenges encountered, and the ways organizations that conduct clinical trials function at an operational level.

Many sponsors developing drugs outsource work to CROs. This means that they do not need as many permanent employees, and can hire specialized personnel to conduct their studies on a trial-by-trial basis. Relationships between sponsors and CROs can take many forms, and the nomenclature used by individual sponsors and CROs can vary. Therefore, you may hear different terms in your own work. However, the general picture painted in this chapter should provide a useful roadmap.

Historically, sponsors often hired CROs to carry out a trial exactly as specified in the study protocol that the sponsors had developed. Additionally, they may have hired several CROs, each fulfilling some of the overall responsibilities of running the trial. In such contexts, the term service provider was appropriate for the CRO. As noted in

Section 1.2.4, this trend is changing, and some sponsors and CROs are establishing relationships that are better described as partnerships, in which sponsors involve CROs early in their clinical development programs and welcome their medical and scientific expertise in the planning and protocol development stages. A single CRO that has provided good consulting at these stages may be given a large role in conducting the trial, or possibly become solely responsible for executing all aspects of the trial. There are mutual benefits should this occur. The sponsor gains additional expertise and economy of services, and the CRO gets more business from a long-term relationship.

4.2 The Outsourcing Process

When a sponsor knows that it will be conducting a clinical trial at some point in the future, and that it wants to hire one or more CROs to run the trial, individuals who specialize in outsourcing prepare a Request for Proposals (RFP). An RFP is typically sent to several CROs along with the respective study protocol. These CROs reply to the RFP by providing (proposing) a detailed plan describing how they would conduct the study and how much they would charge the sponsor for their work. RFPs may be sent first to a relatively small group of CROs that have been carefully selected according to certain performance criteria of particular importance to the sponsor. These CROs are called preferred providers, and they will have signed confidentiality agreements with the sponsor. These agreements are known as Master Service Agreements (MSAs) and sometimes as Non-Disclosure Agreements (NDAs— not to be confused with the same acronym when used to represent a new drug application). This means that the sponsor can send these CROs a study protocol for an upcoming trial secure in the knowledge that their proprietary information will not be shared with other sponsors with whom the CROs may be working.

Outsourcing specialists may perform an initial inspection of the proposals submitted by various CROs, and then (some of) the proposals are forwarded to the study team that has been formed to be in charge of the trial. This team then selects perhaps two or three proposals that look promising, and invites representatives from these CROs to visit their premises for a bid defense. In this meeting the study team asks the CRO representatives many questions, essentially interviewing them in regard to their ability to conduct the trial successfully, and at a price that is acceptable to the sponsor.

4.3 Feasibility Considerations

When an RFP and the associated protocol arrive at a CRO, the documents are channeled directly to the feasibility team. This team's role is to assess the full operational demands of the clinical trial, and to ask (and eventually answer) this question: Can the trial be successfully executed as currently laid out in the protocol? The team initiates a series of investigative process within the CRO that will provide information to help answer the question.

The first step is for a feasibility team member to organize a strategy call, a teleconference involving experts from within the CRO, including, among many others, medics and project managers from the respective therapeutic area. One informative way to evaluate the trial's feasibility is to check past performance metrics for other trials the CRO has successfully completed in the same therapeutic area. Questions of interest include:

- Where were the sites used in the previous trial located?
- How easy was it to recruit and retain the required number of subjects for the previous trial, and did ease of recruitment vary across geographic locations within countries and across countries?
- How similar is the study design on this occasion, including the number of subjects required?

These and other topics will be discussed during the strategy call. Following this call, the feasibility team will usually make one of two decisions:

- It is likely that a few days of additional checking of information will provide a good degree of confidence that the protocol can be executed as currently written.
- A much more extensive evaluative process is needed.

In the later case another six to eight weeks may be needed.

4.3.1 More Extensive Feasibility Evaluations

If the latter decision is made, the feasibility team mobilizes internal and external information-gathering resources. For example, they are likely to create a survey that is sent with the study protocol to physicians in various locations at which the trial may be conducted. The survey asks a series of questions targeted at understanding if the physicians would be able to recruit subjects into the trial and the timeline by which enrollment would be completed.

While waiting to receive feedback from these surveys the feasibility team members continue to mine data from available databases to investigate the prevalence of the disease or clinical condition of concern and to gain a solid understanding of the target patient population that is the focus of the study. Such sites may include prescription and medical claims data bases. Patient advocacy groups for the disease of interest may also be good resources. Consideration of the protocol's inclusion and exclusion criteria is important at this point in estimating how many potential subjects from the overall pool of individuals with the disease would be eligible for enrollment in this particular study as described in the protocol. The goal is to arrive at a realistic estimate of subject availability.

Another aspect in this step-wise evaluative process is to estimate how many other sponsors are currently planning and/or conducting similar trials, and hence 'competing' for the same patients to enroll as subjects. That is, the competitive landscape is of interest. One way to assess this is to go to the web site, www.clinicaltrials.gov, where sponsors are required to register their trials. The CRO may also get information directly from the sponsor sending them the RFP, since many sponsors have 'competitive intelligence' divisions that gather publicly available information on other sponsors' drug pipelines and upcoming likely trials.

When the feasibility team receives back the completed surveys they consider the feedback carefully. From experience, they know that physicians interested in participating in the trial often inflate (unconsciously or consciously) the number of subjects they say they can recruit. They may also make positive statements about the suitability of their facilities and their abilities to operationally execute complicated aspects of the protocol. While such rose-tinted self-appraisals may initially make the physician's site look attractive for inclusion in the trial, subsequent site underperformance has a cascade of unfortunate consequences. Overall subject recruitment is negatively impacted, the sponsor's clinical development program is delayed, and, should the drug eventually be approved for marketing, patients who are prescribed the drug could have benefited from it earlier. Exaggerated claims followed by underperformance can also negatively impact the site, which may never again be considered as a viable option by the CRO (the author has no sympathy in this case: actions have consequences).

4.3.2 Feasibility Reporting

Once the information gathering has been completed, the feasibility team analyzes the data and assimilates the results into a comprehensive report that includes recommendations as to where the study should be conducted, how quickly subjects can be enrolled, and consideration of any potential risks to meeting the enrollment timeline. This report is delivered to the sponsor. Based on their assessment of this information, any causes for concern can be discussed, and the protocol modified to increase the likelihood of the trial's successful and timely execution. The role of feasibility assessments is therefore a critically important one. Their due diligence can preclude the scenario presented at the end of the previous section, and, in contrast, facilitate a successful trial that benefits all concerned.

4.4 Standard Operating Procedures

Like many other organizations, including sponsors, a CRO will have its own standard operating procedures (SOPs). Along with policies, guidelines, and other process-specific documents, SOPs guide everything that the company does. Traditionally, SOPs have been regarded as highly confidential since they are company-specific and capture the essence of a company's operational procedures. More recently, as sponsors and CROs work in partnerships, SOPs may be shared. A question that arises in joint ventures is: In cases where the SOPs that address the same operation differ between sponsor and CRO, which one(s) will be used? There is no fixed answer to this question, since it will vary depending on many factors. However, it is important to ask such questions early in the partnership, and determine the situation-specific answer.

The primary purposes for creating and adhering to SOPs include the following (Spilker, 2009):

- Convey what administrative paperwork must be generated and maintained.
- Help to educate new and current employees on how to perform certain tasks. One of the first tasks you will complete when starting a new job at (or a new position within) a company will be to read general SOPs applicable to the company's general functioning, and others SOPs specific to your job.
- Ensure that repetitive operations are conducted in the same manner each time.
- Convey what testing must be done during various tasks to ensure that they are executed to (or above) the level of quality that meets the expectations of management within the company and external stakeholders.
- Demonstrate to regulatory authorities conducting audits that the company is complying (often stated as 'in compliance') with the requirements of its own SOPs.
- Help to provide protection to the company from law suits.

4.4.1 Balancing the Degree of Flexibility within an SOP

First and foremost, SOPs should be written in a clear, concise, and unambiguous manner. Just how rigid they should be is less certain. This last statement may sound counterintuitive at first: shouldn't these documents specify precisely what should happen in all eventualities? The pragmatic answer is no. A certain degree of rigidity is certainly necessary to ensure that processes operate smoothly, consistently, and reliably within the company. However, SOPs should not be so onerous that their implementation impedes successful work proceeding at a reasonable rate, or so inflexible that, when the company cannot address certain eventualities within the scope of an SOP, they frequently become out of compliance.

4.4.2 Implementing and Maintaining SOPs

When starting a new company and preparing to write the necessary SOPs, the first one should address how to write all subsequent SOPs. It should also state, for example, how new ones are to be approved, how and how frequently existing SOPs are to be reviewed to ensure they are still current and necessary, what the review process will entail, who has ultimate signatory power of approval, and how to ensure that site-specific SOPs (at one location) are not in conflict with company-wide documents (that apply at all company locations world-wide). Maintaining a company's SOPs is no small task, but is a critical one. As Gough and Hamrell (2010) noted, "An SOP is never final until it is retired and the process it supports stops. Each review cycle of active documents is an opportunity to refine and improve processes both for compliance and smooth operations."

4.5 Project Management

Once selected to conduct a specific clinical trial, a CRO has to create its own study team for that trial. This team will include statisticians, investigational site selection specialists, subject recruitment specialists, physicians from the therapeutic area in which the drug falls, clinical trial monitors who will visit the sites and check that the study protocol is being executed correctly, medical monitors who are available to consult on any subject health concerns, data managers and information technology (IT) experts who are responsible for receiving, managing, storing, and integrating the data that will eventually be analyzed and interpreted, and project team leaders or managers who coordinate the efforts of others on the team. In the present context, the term project is used for a drug that is being developed.

Project management is a critical aspect of the clinical trial process whose importance in successful trial execution cannot be overstated. Just a few components of project management include study budgets, timelines, marshalling and distributing resources, appraising metrics on a continual basis, and facilitating communication with all stakeholders. In addition, project managers must conduct their work against a backdrop of tremendous scientific, technical, and financial risks.

4.6 Site and Investigator Recruitment

Site and investigator recruitment is a precursor to the topic of the following section, subject recruitment and retention. However, while they can be meaningfully considered separately, these topics ultimately unify by playing complementary roles in attempting to guarantee the same outcome, i.e., the desired number of subjects completing a sponsor's trial.

4.6.1 Principal Investigators

While there can be exceptions, the vast majority of principal investigators are medical doctors. While this initially may seem entirely appropriate, since physicians comprise the profession that will eventually prescribe a marketed drug to patients, further consideration highlights the paradoxical nature of this arrangement. The essence of a physician's work is to treat every patient as an individual case, tailoring all interventions (pharmaceutical and otherwise) to the unique clinical needs and circumstances of that patient. In contrast, the essence of conducting a clinical trial is to implement a study protocol such that all subjects are (ideally) treated in exactly the same manner, the only difference being which drug treatment they receive. Expressing this more succinctly, conducting a clinical trial is antithetical to clinical practice.

As a general statement, medical schools do not currently provide medical students with a thorough understanding of clinical trial methodology. When this is suggested, a typical reply is that a school's curriculum is already packed with many required courses, and that it is not feasible to consider adding extra classes that could be viewed as adding an extra burden to the students' workload. While not questioning the legitimacy of this argument, a creative solution would undoubtedly be helpful to students who, once practicing medicine, would like to be an investigator for clinical trials. Further discussion of this topic is beyond the scope of this book: the author simply wishes to alert readers to this situation, since there is a great need for well-prepared investigators for future clinical trials.

4.6.2 Responsibilities of Principal Investigators

If a clinical trial is conducted under an IND, each principal investigator (PI) at each investigational site has to sign FDA Form 1572. This is a comprehensive and complex form that, when signed, places legal obligations on the PI to ensure that the trial is conducted as detailed in the form. At larger sites, there may be one or more co-principal investigators (co-PIs) to whom certain responsibilities are delegated. Nonetheless, the PI is still accountable for the conduct of the trial at that site.

4.6.3 Potential Principal Investigators in Private Practice Settings

Physicians in private practice settings who wish to participate in clinical trials for the first time can face a set of challenges not likely to be experienced by colleagues at larger institutions that have been running clinical trials for some time (see the next section). Physicians in these settings may not have a large support system around them that would facilitate the running of clinical trials. Primary motivations for a sponsor when choosing an investigational site and PI include:

- Experience of the PI, and the availability of references from those that can attest to successful performance in previous trials;
- The number of staff present, including study coordinators, nurses, and sub-investigators;
- Experience of the staff;
- The pool of possible subjects who meet the trial's eligibility requirements;
- Evidence that the PI will pay attention to details of the protocol;
- Willingness of the PI to be a team player;
- Offering a competitive budget.

It can be difficult for some potential PIs to meet all of a sponsor's requirements (or desires). This means that the pharmaceutical and biologics industries are losing potentially good sites for largely operational reasons. A new paradigm for success in such settings is discussed in Section 4.10.

4.6.4 Potential Principal Investigators at Larger Medical Institutions

Potential PIs working at large university medical schools or other large medical institutions may find a rich pool of resources available to them. Such centers often have a well-established infrastructure dedicated to facilitating their physicians' participation in clinical trials by providing organizational and personnel support. Many leading institutions have a clinical research center fully staffed by medical, nursing, regulatory, and other essential personnel, thereby providing the support that is much harder for physicians in private practice settings to secure. These clinical research centers can also liaise directly with sponsors to let them know what they offer in terms of therapeutic area expertise, pools of potential subjects, measurement systems already in place, and other features that are likely to facilitate an efficient start-up process for a specific clinical trial.

4.6.5 Principal Investigator Training

While early-phase trials can be conducted at one investigative site, it is much more common to see multicenter trials and hence multiple PIs in Phase III trials. Given that the expertise and previous experiences of these investigators will not be identical, the sponsor must work diligently to enable them all (to the greatest extent possible) to conduct every aspect of the trial in the standardized manner detailed in the study's protocol. Examples of areas in which PIs, and their study staff, may need training include:

- Accurate implementation of inclusion/exclusion criteria such that (only) subjects who are appropriate for the trial are enrolled;
- Fully understanding (and accepting) the need for adherence to all study protocol procedures;
- Understanding current Good Clinical Practice (cGCP);
- Completing case report forms (CRFs) accurately and completely, and how to make (and document) changes if and when necessary;
- Collecting, processing, storing, and shipping any biological samples (e.g., blood and urine) in a uniform manner;
- Diagnosing and rating the nature and severity of adverse events, and particularly adverse events of special interest, accurately and in a uniform manner across all sites;
- Reporting these adverse events uniformly across all sites;
- Developing strategies for communication between sites and the sponsor (and the CRO representing the sponsor).

Various strategies exist for implementing investigator training. One option is for all investigators to attend a training session called an Investigator Meeting (IM), run by the CRO or possibly by a professional training organization on behalf of the CRO. In trials for which the sites are in close proximity, it may be logistically possible to run just one meeting. However, in the case of multi-center Phase III trials the sites may be spread across a country, and even across various continents. It may therefore be advantageous to run several meetings. In this case, attention must be paid to standardizing the training course itself. Having the same trainers running multiple meetings is ideal, but when the investigators speak many different languages this can be a considerable challenge.

An alternative option is for the trainers to visit each site to conduct training. As in the previous strategy, more sites and greater geographical diversity makes this potentially more challenging. At one time, it was considered somewhat of a 'perk' for investigators to attend such meetings, since they were often held at luxurious settings in exotic locations. This is much less the case now. Additionally, some potential investigators would much rather have trainers come to visit them, since this is more time efficient for their busy schedules.

A third strategy is running web-based meetings. This can involve training modules that investigators and their staff must complete, and also interactive web-based sessions, potentially using video capabilities as well as just on-screen materials. Whichever method is chosen by the sponsor and/or their CRO, the more thorough the training, the more likely it is that investigators and their staff will implement the study protocol correctly.

4.7 Subject Recruitment and Retention
Jaishankar (2009) commented as follows:

> [Subject] recruitment and retention remains one of the most significant challenges faced by the pharmaceutical industry today...As recruiting becomes more diverse and complex, pharmaceutical companies are striving to discover new innovative ways to facilitate recruitment and keep [subjects] enrolled in the clinical

trial. With more and more clinical trials being done on a global level, it is imperative to have an understanding of both government regulations and social protocol that accompany these new markets. (p. 26)

4.7.1 Subject Recruitment

While individual investigators can play an important role in subject recruitment—their access to potential subjects likely having been a reason for their being selected to participate in the trial—the primary responsibility for subject recruitment falls squarely on the sponsor. Creation and implementation of a recruitment strategy and plan is a critical operational step. This plan should be a formal written document that carefully considers best-case and worst-case scenarios, takes into account various timing influences (e.g., national holiday periods, seasons of the year, likely onset of flu season), and has contingencies built in to address all anticipated potential recruitment barriers.

The following operational definition of recruitment is useful:
- Identifying potential pools of subjects and specific individual subjects who may be eligible to enroll in the trial;
- Attracting those individuals to consider participation;
- Discussing the trial with them;
- Prescreening subjects;
- Having subjects read an informed consent form, answering any questions they may have, and then having the subjects sign the consent form;
- Conducting a more complete and formal screening procedure;
- Being able to state that subjects are now enrolled in the trial.

Recruitment is of ongoing interest to a sponsor throughout a trial, and there are several common metrics addressing this. One is 'first subject first visit,' the date on which the first subject completes his or her first visit to the investigational site (there will typically be many visits spread over a period of time as detailed in the study protocol.) Another is the date when 50% of the sites have each enrolled at least one subject.

Traditional subject recruitment strategies include the following:
- Advertisements on radio and television, and in print media;
- Mailing flyers to individuals and patient advocacy groups;
- Data mining from insurance company databases;
- Using web sites to publicize the trial;
- Posting information on a hospital's bulletin board;
- Hospital staff wearing lapel pins that bring attention to the trial.

Cabell (2009) discussed another approach that focuses on understanding and utilizing the 'patient pathway,' the route by which patients receive treatment. By understanding and documenting the pathway via which patients with the disease or condition of clinical concern of interest receive their medical care, it becomes possible for recruitment specialists to reach out to clinicians and other health care professionals who provide the care. This allows the specialists to access the appropriate patients and, should they be willing, recruit them as subjects for the trial.

4.7.2 Subject Retention

It has become widely accepted that sponsors need to devote considerable resources to subject retention as well as recruitment: the ultimate goal is for an enrolled subject to complete participation in the trial, not just start participation in it. Many characteristics of a subject's participation in the trial can influence the likelihood that he or she will complete the trial, including:

- The length of the treatment period. Subjects have personal and professional lives, and events that preclude trial completion, e.g., personal or family illness, relocating, financial difficulties, do and will happen. Some trials have relatively long treatment periods, and the sponsor cannot alter this, but the length should alert the sponsor to the need for appropriate contingency plans.
- How onerous participation is. If the trial's protocol requires subjects to undergo many procedures at many visits, with-

drawal rate may increase. The burden of the trial should be considered at the protocol development phase, with an eye to decreasing non-critical subject tasks, such as filling out a large number of questionnaires that do not address the primary objective. Another potentially influential factor is the method of drug administration. While the majority of small-molecule investigational drugs are administered orally, injection is typical for biologics. Some individuals (the author included) do not like needles.

- Ease of traveling to the site. If many subjects participating at a given site have to travel a considerable distance, and/or at considerable expense, each time they visit the site, the sponsor is well advised to address this proactively.

Specific retention strategies include:

- Providing reimbursement for expenses such as parking, meals, and baby-sitting;
- Calling subjects shortly before each visit to remind them of the visit and to assure them that provisions for their attendance are in place;
- Paying for, or actually providing transportation to and from the site;
- Providing escorts from and back to a parking lot, particularly if it is not well lit, and/or in bad weather;
- Optimizing the environment in the subject waiting area. This can include having sufficient and appropriately current magazines, providing toys for children who accompany subjects out of necessity, and ensuring that all trial staff treat the subjects and accompanying family members courteously at all times.
- Reminding the subjects throughout the trial that their participation is extremely valuable in developing a drug that, if approved, may provide considerable benefit to many patients. This can be done verbally and also by sending out regular newsletters.

4.8 Monitoring Clinical Trials

Monitoring a clinical trial is essential in the acquisition of optimum quality data. Monitoring is traditionally performed by individuals with titles such as clinical research associates (CRAs), clinical research monitors (CRMs), and medical monitors. Monitors have responsibilities before the trial starts and throughout its implementation. Preliminary visits to sites enable relationships with investigators and their colleagues to be established and training to be conducted. Also, before the trial commences, the monitor will go through an extensive pretrial checklist to ensure, for example, that initial supplies of the drug products have arrived, any electronic data capture (eDC) equipment to be used is installed and tested, and informed consent forms and procedural manuals are available. Critical issues that need monitoring during the trial include recruiting and retaining subjects and investigators, checking on protocol compliance by both subjects and investigators, performing a quality control function by overseeing the collection of data on the CRFs, evaluating adherence to the trial's treatment regimens, and limiting adverse events.

Traditionally, monitors have visited investigational sites at regular intervals throughout the trial. A new model for monitoring is discussed in Chapter 5.

4.9 Underperforming and Non-performing Clinical Trial Sites

Once a site has been selected for a clinical trial, there will be an expectation that the site recruits and enrolls a certain number of subjects in a certain timeframe, and a similar expectation that a certain number will complete their participation by a certain date. However, the performance metrics for both are extremely concerning.

While precise quantification of the length and expense of the entire process of new drug development (including nonclinical research) is difficult, it is sufficient to note that respective values of 10-15 years and US$1.3 billion are realistic and informative approximations at the time of this book's publication. Precise quantification is equally difficult when examining site performance across the entire biopharmaceutical industry, partly because some sponsors are less forthcoming with such information than others. However, once again, realistic approximations can informatively be made, and the figures presented here are done so in this spirit. Consider the following:

- More than 70% of physician investigator sites are under-performing or non-performing when conducting clinical trials;
- More than 80% fail to enroll subjects on time;
- 30% fail to enroll a single subject;
- 80% of subjects who complete the trial do so at 20% of the sites (the so-called '80-20 rule');
- 70% of physician investigators who take part in their first trial do not wish to participate in another trial.

Examples of the consequences of these metrics include the following:

- New drug development is excessively costly, since a lot of time, effort, and money is completely wasted.
- New drug applications to regulatory agencies are delayed, resulting in delayed time to market for approved drugs.
- In cases of unmet medical needs, and when a drug is much better than its already-marketed competitors, patients have to wait longer to receive beneficial therapy.
- Delayed time to market costs a sponsor a lot of money (the figure of US$1 million per day is sometimes quoted).

Additionally, consider further the metric that 70% of physician investigators who take part in their first trial do not wish to participate in another trial. Several inferences can be made from this. First, if physician investigators are so disappointed (frustrated, distracted, annoyed) by their experiences that they do not want to take part in another trial, it could reasonably be argued that the quality of care the physician was able to provide to their patients during the time of their involvement in the trial—which, after all, is their number one priority—may not have been what the physician would normally have provided. (Note: This is absolutely no criticism, stated or implied, of physicians: comments here relate solely to the difficulties experienced by caring and skilled clinicians trying their best to fulfill both clinical trial and patient care responsibilities in the current environment of clinical trial execution at investigator sites.)

Second, while clinical trials are totally separate from clinical care (a point noted several times already), participating in a clinical trial can bring additional medical focus to subjects. Subjects frequently receive free medical examinations as part of a study protocol, examinations that they may not be able to afford normally if they have inadequate (or no) health insurance. The ethical principle of justice requires that the burdens and benefits of participation in clinical trials are distributed evenly and fairly. It is possible that caring physicians who practice in under-served communities, and who wish to do everything possible for their patients—including providing them with the opportunity to be subjects in clinical trials and therefore to have access to potentially life-saving new therapies—may find being an investigator particularly burdensome since they do not have the resources of colleagues in other medical settings.

4.9.1 Limitations of the Current Model

While neither sponsors nor investigators are happy with these performance metrics, the current model imposes certain constraints that preclude certain changes. Foremost among these are legal and potential conflict-of-interest concerns. Neither sponsors nor the CROs with whom they are working (partnering) can operationally manage the physician offices acting as investigational sites and the physician personnel conducting the trials because of these conflict-of-interest issues. One potential solution tried by CROs has been to set up 'firewalls' and assign clinical research coordinators (CRCs) to physicians' offices. However, these CRCs have typically not been trained in the systems required to ensure operational efficiencies.

A new model that addresses these limitations is described in the following section.

4.10 The Site-specific CRO

At this point, it is appropriate to introduce two new terms. First, the CROs that we have discussed up to here can be thought of as Sponsor CROs: their responsibility is to their drug development partner, their sponsor. The second term is Site-specific CRO (SS-CRO). An SS-CRO partners with the physician's office and the physician who is the principal investigator at that site. Their responsibility is therefore quite different from that of the (traditional) Sponsor CRO: SS-CROs work for, and partner with, physician's offices and focus on optimizing operational quality at that site (see www.ctmginc.com).

An SS-CRO therefore functions as a business associate of the physician office, planning and implementing cGMP-like processes at physician investigator sites under tight quality control and quality assurance. The SS-CRO's personnel work with, and at, the physician site to ensure all necessary operational knowledge is imported, and operational excellence is attained. This model means that physician investigators can focus on three things for which they are eminently well trained—the clinical care of the patients in their practice, the medical requirements of the study protocol, and ensuring subjects' safety while participating in the trial.

CHAPTER 5

Information-driven Clinical Trials

5.1 Introduction

PRECEDING CHAPTERS HAVE discussed the acquisition of optimum quality clinical trial data. It was noted in Section 1.3 that the anatomy of a clinical trial can be represented by a model comprising three components:

- Study design: It is critical to use a design that will facilitate the collection of required data.
- Trial conduct: This comprises employing optimum quality experimental methodology and optimum quality operational execution. The former means that optimum quality data *can* be collected, and the latter ensures that such data *are indeed* collected.
- Analysis of the data collected and interpretation of these analyses in the context of the research question the trial has been designed to answer.

Data are of critical importance, but it is their translation into information, and the use of this information as the rational basis for decision-making, that is the ultimate goal. Brown Stafford (2011) described the following sequence of steps in this context:

Data » Data analytics » Expert interpretation »
Information » Decision-making

This chapter first describes the traditional data management model, and then discusses a model that transitions to the 'management of information' in a (near) real-time manner, demonstrating how the power and applicability of information technology is of tremendous benefit in the drug development process.

5.2 The Case Report Form

Case report forms (CRFs) are used to record data collected during a trial. They record all of the information specified in the study protocol for each subject (all data recorded on the CRF must be verifiable from original source documentation). While the traditional paper CRF format is still used, electronic data collection (eDC) is becoming more common. It is helpful to utilize eDC when possible, since eDC at the time of the subject's clinic visits and/or procedures makes the data entry process quicker and less susceptible to error. It also offers the chance to monitor data collection in a timely manner as the clinical trial progresses, which facilitates the opportunity to detect trends toward poor quality or unexpected data that may be the result of the investigator site failing to adhere to the protocol. Early detection and correction of such issues is much preferable to the alternative.

The following points can be made regarding the purpose, design, and nature of CRFs:

- Well-designed CRFs capture all essential scientific and regulatory information and do not capture information that is not needed. Collected data include those related to study endpoints, adverse events, potential confounding influences, and protocol compliance.
- Their design benefits considerably from involvement by those who will record information on them and statisticians who will eventually be analyzing the data.
- They should be clear, easy to read, and able to be completed quickly and efficiently and capture data unambiguously.
- Good CRFs are designed according to the specific trial's requirements. Do not start by simply deciding to use the data collection forms that were used in previous studies. If there are some

questions on previous forms that address the collection of data you need, can those questions be improved?

- CRFs should be designed to collect the data needed and only the data needed. That is, create data collection forms that provide data that will address the objectives of the study and only those objectives. Collecting additional data is unnecessarily wasteful of time, money, and resources.

It is important to create a cross-functional team to design a CRF that is clear, easily completed by investigators, and efficient for data management and statistical analysis processes.

5.3 Data Management Plans

A Data Management Plan for a clinical trial is written along with the study protocol and statistical analysis plan before the study commences. It identifies the documentation that will be produced as a result of all of the data collected during the conduct of the trial, who will be responsible for collecting the data, and which standard operating procedures (SOPs) will govern these activities. Topics typically covered by the plan include:

- Design of the CRF;
- Entering data;
- Cleaning the data;
- Managing laboratory data;
- Serious adverse event data handling;
- Creating data reports;
- Transferring data;
- Quality assurance processes that will be implemented to ensure that all data management procedures are compliant with regulatory governance.

The quality assurance component is vital. While differing definitions of quality activities can be found, one way to think about these activities is to regard quality assurance (QA) as a process involving the prevention, detection, and correction of errors or problems, and quality control (QC) as a check of the process. The data stored in the database need to be complete and accurate. Processes that check data and correct them where necessary (i.e., make a change to the database) need to be formalized, and all corrections documented in an audit trail such that a later audit can reveal exactly how the final database was created.

5.4 Data Management

Data management is an important intermediary between data acquisition, the province of experimental methodology and operational execution, and data analysis. Various kinds of data are collected during the conduct of a clinical trial. A brief list of clinical data (numerical representations of biological information collected from the subjects participating in the trial) includes the following: age, height, weight, and sex; questionnaire data concerning a multitude of topics; physiological measurements made before, during, and possibly after the treatment period; adverse events reported (adverse events are discussed in the following chapter); images from various imaging techniques; and laboratory data representing the results of assays for various body fluid samples (e.g., blood and urine) taken from subjects at many points during the trial. The data for each individual subject are linked to a unique subject identifier rather than his or her name. Other data collected pertain to operational aspects of the trial. For example, information on subject recruitment and retention rates, the timely delivery (or not) of study drugs to the investigational sites, protocol deviations (by investigators and subjects), and data quality are all of interest.

Many data that are collected can now be fed directly from the measuring instrument to computer databases, thereby avoiding the potential of human data entry error. However, this is not universally true. Therefore, careful strategies have been developed to scrutinize data as they are entered. The double-entry method requires that each data set is entered twice (usually by different operators) and that these entries are compared by a computer for any discrepancies. This method operates on the premise that two identical errors are probabilistically very unlikely, and, therefore, that every time the two entries match the data are correct. In contrast, dissimilar entries are identified, the source (original) data located, and the correct data point confirmed.

To facilitate the eventual statistical analysis of the enormous amount of data acquired during a clinical trial, recording and maintaining these data are critical requirements. Database development, implementation, and maintenance therefore require attention. The goals of a database are to store data in a manner that facilitates prompt retrieval while not diminishing their security or integrity.

There are several types of database models. Clinical research typically utilizes one of two types, the flat file database or the relational database. The flat file database model is simple but restrictive, and it becomes less easy to use as the amount of data stored increases. This model can also lead to data redundancy (the same information, e.g., a subject's birth date, being entered multiple times) and consequently to potential errors. This model works well for relatively small databases.

Relational databases are more flexible, but they can be complex, and careful initial work is needed. This work involves initial logical modeling of the database. The defining feature of a relational database is that data are stored in tables, and these tables can be related to each other. This reduces data redundancy. Subject identifiers in one table, for example, can be related to their heights in another table, their baseline blood pressure in another table, and so on, thereby eliminating the need to store identifiers with each individual set of measurements. Since these databases can contain huge amounts of tables, use of one of several commercially available relational database management systems is typical.

5.5 From Data to Information

As noted in Section 5.1, Brown Stafford (2011) described the following sequence of steps:

Data » Data analytics » Expert interpretation
» Information » Decision-making

Implicit in this sequence is the conceptual and practical evolution from data management to information management. Data and their successful management lead to a wealth of information that also needs managing successfully. When this is done, as noted at the start of this chapter, the information provides the rational basis for decision-making during a drug's clinical development program.

Many decisions during drug development concern whether or not to proceed to the next step in the process (e.g., moving from completion of Phase II trials to the commencement of Phase III trials). Such decisions are commonly referred to as 'go/no-go' decisions. Adequate evidence needs to be obtained, and documented, to permit careful consideration of the pros and cons of proceeding. Given a finite amount of resources and, particularly in the case of larger biopharmaceutical companies, a choice of drug candidates upon which to focus these resources, it is financially prudent for them to proceed only if there is a reasonable chance of success (the definition of 'reasonable' being unique to each sponsor and drug candidate). While business driven, the choice to pursue development programs that are likely to yield successful drugs is also in the best interests of patients: Pursuing development plans for drug candidates that are likely to fail would reduce the sponsor's ability to work on drugs that may get approved and help patients. Other decisions are made during the conduct of an individual trial, as discussed in Section 5.7.1 and 5.7.2.

5.6 Innovations to Advance Information Management

Brown Stafford (2011) discussed innovations to advance information management, including:

- Technology: Integrated data in real time;
- Process: A new operating model.

5.6.1 Integrated Data in Real Time

Advances in information technology now permit integrated data to be available much more quickly than was previous possible, in a real-time manner. The tremendous range and extent of data collected in a clinical trial was noted in the previous section. While any individual data set can be informative in isolation, being able to examine integrated data in real time allows better insights to be gained during a trial's conduct. Reviewing the cumulative data acquired at any point in time is particularly informative. For example, the identification of safety issues may be greatly enhanced by having a multi-parameter integrated data set to inspect. If several biological parameters are showing relatively small but consistently concerning changes, the identification of such a pattern may be of considerable significance in protecting the health and safety of the subjects participating in the trial.

5.6.2 Process Innovation: Data-driven Triggered Monitoring

The monitoring of clinical trials was discussed in Section 4.8. More accurately, the traditional model of monitoring trials was discussed, one in which monitors made regular and costly trips to investigational sites. The ability to monitor real-time integrated data (and hence information) allows triggered monitoring to address various issues, including:

- Subject safety issues
- Recruitment and retention
- Data quality issues
- Protocol deviations

Such triggered monitoring is more cost-effective and efficient than the old model described in Section 4.8.

5.7 Technology-enabled Trials: Reducing Time-to-Market

New drug development is a lengthy, expensive, and complex endeavor. While this book has focused on clinical trials, considerable time and expenditure is spent before clinical trials commence on the drug's nonclinical development program and, before that, the processes of drug discovery. As noted in Section 4.9, reasonable estimates for the time and money spent from the beginning of the drug discovery process to the time a new drug receives marketing approval are 10-15 years and US$1.3 billion. Not surprisingly, therefore, there is enormous interest among many stakeholders in the biopharmaceutical and healthcare industries in reducing this time and financial expenditure. Given our focus on clinical trials, initiatives to reduce the time taken during a drug's clinical development program are of immediate interest.

Enhanced data capture capabilities, enabled by advances in information technology, are making more accurate and integrated information available more quickly to drug developers. This allows better decisions to be made at earlier times. As noted earlier, eDC systems collect data electronically directly from an investigational site. In addition, data integration tools combine electronic data from various sources in real time. Another beneficial component is the work of the Clinical Data Interchange Standards Consortium (CDISC: see www.cdisc.org). Their standards initiatives have created new opportunities to streamline the clinical research process.

5.7.1 Adaptive Trials

The traditional study design model for clinical trials is the fixed design, one in which there is no latitude to deviate from the precise plans detailed in the study protocol and the associated statistical analysis plan. The study design is thus specified at the beginning of the trial, the number of subjects that will be enrolled is clearly stated, and the plan for data analysis is laid out in detail before the trial starts. Once the trial has commenced, it progresses as planned until its conclusion. All of the data are collected together, and "database lock" occurs. Statistical analyses are then conducted as detailed in the study protocol and/or statistical analysis plan. Consider a multi-center Phase III trial involving 3,000 subjects (half randomized to the drug treatment group and the other half randomized to the placebo treatment group). The time span from the 'first subject first visit' to the 'last subject last visit' may well be several years, even though each subject's participation might only be several months in duration: Since not all subjects commence their participation at the same time, the duration of the trial will likely be much longer than the duration of the treatment. Once all data are assembled for database lock, it will still take some time for the analyses to be conducted, and so the results of the trial will not be known for several years after the trial's commencement.

In contrast, adaptive designs have inherent flexibility to be modified in midstream following inspection of data collected to date. Your initial reaction to this might be that it sounds a bit like cheating: Having knowledge of the data collected to date and the ability to modify the study design based on that knowledge introduces a degree of subjectivity into what is purportedly an objective process. If so, your reaction is a legitimate one. Fortunately, ethical and scientific procedures are put in place at the beginning of adaptive trials to maintain the validity and integrity of the trial, and hence the integrity and usefulness of the trial's results.

Interim analyses are analyses conducted during a trial, using the data that have been collected up to that point in time. In adaptive trials, the purpose of the interim analyses is to determine how best to modify the remainder of the trial to increase the amount of useful information that can be gained from the trial. A data monitoring process is necessary to facilitate interim analysis (this is a different use of the term monitoring from that used for the role of a monitor who checks on the quality and accuracy of data collected from specific investigational sites). Data monitoring in this context is conducted by a multidisciplinary group of individuals who are called a Data Monitoring Committee, a Data and Safety Monitoring Board, or one of several other similar names. Interim monitoring of accumulating data is critical to the ethics (including protecting the safety of participating subjects), efficiency, integrity, and credibility of the trial and its conclusions.

Before an adaptive trial starts, a Charter is written and agreed upon by the trial's sponsor and the committee. This describes the structure and operation of the committee and specifies its activities and responsibilities. The committee typically has access to the data collected to date in an unblinded manner. That is, they will have knowledge of which subjects received the drug and which received the placebo, knowledge that is deliberately not available to the investigators conducting the trial or to the subjects participating in it (recall discussions in Section 3.2.2). Once the statistician(s) on the committee have conducted the interim analysis, an interim report is prepared, which guides any modifications made to the rest of the trial.

For additional discussion of adaptive trials, see Rosenberg (2010).

5.7.2 Group Sequential Trials

Interim analyses are also performed in group sequential trials. Like adaptive trials, these also differ from the traditional fixed design trial. In this case, the maximum number of subjects that may complete the trial is specified in the study protocol (which is equivalent to the statement of subjects who will complete a fixed design trial). However, interim analyses are planned at various stages throughout the trial's execution.

Consider again a Phase III trial involving 3,000 subjects. It might be the case that an interim analysis is planned once 500 subjects (approximately 250 in the drug treatment group and 250 in the placebo treatment group) have completed their participation. The purpose of the interim analyses is to determine if the trial should be terminated at that point. Reasons for termination would be that the data collected to date already demonstrate in a compelling manner that the drug is effective and safe, or that it is toxic. Another reason is called termination for futility. In that case, it is determined that, even if the trial went all the way to its maximum size (the maximum number of subjects completed the trial), the data collected would not be able to provide meaningful evidence for decision-making.

In this example, if the trial were not terminated, it would continue until another 'group' of 500 subjects had completed their participation, and then the analyses would be repeated on the data collected from all 1,000 subjects. This procedure continues until the trial is terminated due to the results of one of the series of interim analyses, or until all 3,000 subjects have completed the trial. Because it is possible that multiple sets of analyses will be conducted, with a maximum number of six sets if the trial proceeds all the way to its maximum size, sophisticated statistical procedures have to be implemented to address the issue of multiple comparisons: These need not be addressed here, but it is important to note that they must be used.

CHAPTER 6

Assessment of Safety

6.1 Introduction

THE SAFETY OF a drug is addressed at all stages in its life history. This starts long before the drug is administered to humans during clinical trials: By the time Phase I trials commence the sponsor will have collected considerable amounts of safety data during the nonclinical development program. Safety will be assessed throughout the preapproval clinical development program, and, if the drug is approved for marketing, it will be assessed throughout the time the drug is on the market. As in other chapters, the focus here is on Phase III trials.

Given the tremendous importance of drug safety, it may come as somewhat of a surprise that the analysis of safety data from Phase III trials is not particularly sophisticated. Historically, safety data have been presented descriptively in regulatory submissions. This is in stark contrast to the analysis of efficacy data, which is rigorously defined and based on inferential statistical analysis, as discussed in the following chapter. This situation has now changed for some specific safety data (see Caveney and Turner, 2010; Salvi et al, 2010; Turner and Caveney, 2010; Satin et al, 2011), and may change for other safety data in the future.

6.2 Providing Safety Data to Prescribing Physicians and Patients

Jumping ahead for a while to the point where a drug has recently been approved, consider a scenario in which a prescribing physician is discussing with a patient whether this drug is a good treatment option for the patient (therapeutic decisions are ideally made by a 'health team' comprising the physician and the patient). What kinds of safety-related information might the doctor and the patient find useful? Examples include:

- How likely is the patient to experience an adverse drug reaction? (The term adverse drug reaction is employed once the drug is on the market. Before that point, as will be seen shortly, the term adverse event is used in clinical trials.)
- Are the typical adverse drug reactions temporary or permanent in nature?
- How likely is the patient to suffer an adverse drug reaction that is extremely serious, or even life-threatening?
- How might the risk of an adverse drug reaction vary with different doses of the drug?
- How might the risk of an adverse drug reaction change with increasing length of treatment?
- Are there any specific clinical parameters that should be monitored more closely than usual in patients receiving this drug?

When a drug is first marketed, the best available information upon which a doctor and patient can form answers to such questions is the safety information gathered during preapproval clinical trials. This information is provided in the drug's package insert or label. The content of the label will have been discussed by the sponsor and the regulatory agency granting marketing approval, and eventually the label is approved by the agency. It includes the best available data about the drug's safety at that point in time.

6.3 The Clinical Study Report

Clinical trial data, both safety and efficacy, are typically presented in a Clinical Study Report (CSR) that is suitable for submission to a regulatory agency. Each CSR has various sections, including subject demographics and accountability, safety data, and efficacy data. The first two of these are addressed in this section, and, as noted previously, efficacy is discussed in the following chapter.

6.3.1 Subject Demographics and Accountability

Describing, or summarizing, the tremendous amount of data that are collected in a clinical trial is typically a useful first step in reporting the results of the trial. Simple descriptors such as the total number of subjects in the trial, the numbers of subjects that received the drug treatment and the placebo treatment, respectively, information concerning sex (male and female) and ethnicity (e.g., Caucasian, African American, Latino), the average age of the subjects in each treatment group, and baseline data of relevance (e.g., weight, blood pressure, and heart rate) help to set the scene for more detailed reporting. Information concerning the use of concomitant or concurrent medications and evaluations of subject adherence or compliance with the trial's treatment schedule is also typically presented.

This information can be usefully summarized in in-text tables that are placed in the body of the text in CSRs. In each case, the source of the information presented must be cited. The source is typically one of many listings that are appended to the report. Listings are comprehensive lists that provide all information collected during the trial.

Table 6.1 provides an example of an in-text table from a hypothetical clinical trial that summarizes subject accountability.

Table 6.1: Subject Accountability (Clinical Trial 123XYZ)

	Number (%) of Subjects	
	Drug (*N*=200)	Placebo (*N*=200)
Completion Status		
Completed study	160 (80)	180 (90)
Withdrew prematurely	40 (20)	20 (10)
Premature Withdrawals		
Adverse event	20 (10)	6 (3)
Withdrew consent	10 (5)	4 (2)
Protocol violation	10 (5)	8 (4)
Other	0	2 (1)

Other: 1. [Description of reason]. 2. [Description or reason] Source Table: ABC

Several comments about these hypothetical data, deliberately chosen to make the math easy, are appropriate. First, it is possible but unlikely that the numbers of subjects for the two treatment groups would be identical in a real study. Presenting percentages as well as absolute numbers is therefore useful, since the percentages allow for differing totals of subjects in each group. Second, the numbers of subjects in the individual categories must add up to the respective group totals. Third, explanation of (any) other reasons for premature withdrawal should be presented, either in text form above or below the table or in footnote form immediately underneath the table.

6.3.2 Adverse Events

General safety assessments are wide-ranging, and, as noted, are typically presented descriptively. Safety-related data can be considered at four levels: extent of exposure to the drug; adverse events; laboratory tests; and vital signs. We will focus on adverse events (AEs).

During the course of a clinical trial it is likely that many subjects will have some form of AEs. The longer the study and the sicker the subjects are, the more AEs there will likely be. When reporting the results from the clinical trial, therefore, it is of interest to know about the frequency of all adverse events. Several different kinds of adverse events can be distinguished:

- Pretreatment adverse events;
- Treatment adverse events;
- Drug-related adverse events;
- Serious adverse events (SAEs);
- Adverse events of special interest;
- Adverse events leading to withdrawal from the study.

There are various ways to provide this information, including listings and in-text summary tables.

Descriptive statistics for AEs typically include rates of occurrence of the events in exposed groups overall and among sub-groups of subjects (e.g., according to age and sex) to look for any potential patterns of differential rates of adverse events.

Typically, a sponsor will report adverse events that occurred in at least a given percentage of the subjects in either group. Data for both treatment groups employed will be provided for any AE listed for either group. Data are often presented in descending order of occurrence. Similar presentations of these data are included in the labels of marketed drugs.

CHAPTER 7

Assessment of Efficacy

7.1 Introduction

FOR REGULATORY AGENCIES to decide that a drug should be approved for marketing, the sponsor needs to provide compelling evidence of efficacy. The discipline of Statistics enables provision of such evidence by using procedures that everyone has agreed to honor: If the results of a Phase III trial attain statistical significance, all stakeholders have previously agreed that such results provide compelling evidence of efficacy. (In many cases, statistically significant evidence of efficacy from two independently conducted Phase III trials is required, but the points of importance in this chapter can be made by considering a single trial.)

However, this is just the first step in a two-step evaluation process. The second step is the evaluation of the drug's clinical significance: That is, does the trial provide compelling evidence of clinically significant efficacy? If a regulatory agency decides that there is compelling evidence of both statistical significance and clinical significance, and if they also decide that the drug's safety profile is acceptable when considered in conjunction with its efficacy, the agency will approve the drug for marketing.

7.2 Making Inferences from a Single Clinical Trial

The ultimate purpose of the results from a clinical trial is not to tell us precisely what happened in that trial, but, in combination with results from other trials in the drug's clinical development program, to gain insight into likely drug responses in patients who would be prescribed the drug should it be approved for marketing. This is a fundamental concept in assessments of both safety and efficacy. The data from a given trial, i.e., from a given set of subjects who participated in the trial, can be used to infer what is likely to be the case for patients who are prescribed the marketed drug in the future. To facilitate such inference, one branch of the discipline of Statistics, inferential statistics, is employed. A strict set of analytical strategies allows such inference to be made, allowing the results to be considered as a meaningful indication of likely responses in a much greater number of patients who may be prescribed the drug in the future.

Consider a single clinical trial in which we assess the changes in MAP (mean arterial pressure) in two groups of subjects, one receiving the drug of interest and the other receiving placebo. (Recalling the terms learned earlier in the book, this is a randomized, double-blind, controlled, parallel-groups study design.) While MAP (like all other parameters) has a unit of measurement, i.e., mmHg, we will leave this out of our discussion for now so that we can focus on the values themselves.

We wish to calculate the drug's treatment effect in this trial. This treatment effect can be defined as follows: Mean change from baseline MAP to end-of-treatment MAP in the drug treatment group minus mean change from baseline MAP to end-of-treatment MAP in the placebo treatment group. (As noted earlier, even though the placebo is not pharmacologically active it is typically the case that subjects in the placebo treatment group will show small changes in MAP across the trial.) Imagine that the mean change for the drug treatment group is an decrease of 8.00, and the mean change for the placebo treatment group is a decrease of 1.00. The treatment effect is therefore calculated as 8.00 minus 1.00, i.e., 7.00. Including the units of measurement, the drug's treatment effect is 7.00 mmHg.

This result is the precise answer for the data acquired from the subjects in this single clinical trial. However, as just noted, our primary interest lies with obtaining an informed estimate of responses that would likely be seen in the general population of patients if the drug is approved. In contrast to the precisely known treatment effect obtained from the subject sample that participated in the trial, the true treatment effect for the population of interest is unknown. Therefore, we wish to use the known treatment effect from the trial, along with all of the individual data that led to the treatment effect's calculation, to provide a meaningful estimate of the true but unknown population treatment effect. When referring to this process of informed estimation of the population treatment effect, the treatment effect from the trial is now called the treatment effect point estimate: it is a single value (a point on a numerical scale), and it is an estimate of the true but unknown population treatment effect.

The next step is to place a confidence interval around this treatment effect point estimate. The details of the calculation of confidence intervals are not necessary here, and the example is presented conceptually. A confidence interval (CI) consists of a lower limit, which will lie below the point estimate, and an upper limit that lies above the point estimate. This form of confidence interval thus has two 'sides.' They are calculated by subtracting and adding the same value from and to the treatment effect point estimate:

Limits of a two-sided CI = Treatment effect point estimate $\pm$ X

where X is a number that is calculated using every value collected from the two treatment groups.

Three commonly used confidence intervals are the two-sided 90% CI, the two-sided 95% CI, and the two-sided 99% CI: we will use the two-sided 95% CI in our examples. In the scenario of interest here, these limits will lie equidistantly around the point estimate since, as just noted, they are calculated by subtracting and adding the same value from and to the treatment effect point estimate. Between the lower limit and the upper limit there is a range of values. In this context, a confidence interval is a range of values that is likely to cover the true but unknown population treatment effect. For the 95% CI we can make the following statement:

- The two-sided 95% CI placed around the treatment effect point estimate is a range of values that we are 95% confident will cover the true but unknown population treatment effect.

7.3 Statistically Significant Efficacy

Consider these hypothetical data from a randomized, controlled, parallel-groups Phase III clinical trial of a new antihypertensive drug. The total number of subjects used in this example is just 21, an extremely unrealistic number: an actual trial of this kind may have 3000-5000 subjects. Nonetheless, this very small dataset can be used to illustrate the key points. You will notice that the number of subjects in the two groups is not identical. While it is statistically advantageous for the numbers of subjects in the treatment groups to be as similar as possible, in practice it is unlikely that they will be identical. The following hypothetical data represent decreases in MAP from baseline to the end of the treatment period:

- Drug treatment group (N=10): 3, 0, 3, 8, 5, 9, 4, 7, 5, 6.
- Placebo treatment group (N=11): 4, 2, 2, 0, 1, 0, 1, 4, 3, 2, 3.

A statistical analysis called the independent-groups t-test can be used to analyze these data. The term independent-groups reflects the fact that the two treatment groups comprise different individuals (independent-groups analyses are used for data from parallel-groups studies). Like many inferential statistical analyses used to evaluate efficacy, this t-test results in two values. The first is called a test statistic, and the second is an associated probability value, i.e., a p-value. The name t-test is used since the test statistic provided by this test is called t.

Cutting straight to the chase, conducting the independent-groups t-test on these data provides the following test statistic:

$$t(19) = 3.27$$

The number 19 (the Degrees of Freedom associated with the test statistic) is two less than the total of subjects in both groups, which we have already noted is 21. Many times when results are presented in CSRs and publications in medical journals the Degrees of Freedom are omitted, but nonetheless they are vital components of the methodology used to determine the final result from the statistical test. (Degrees of Freedom are not covered in detail here: More discussion of this topic will be provided in Volume 2 of this series, entitled *Introduction to Design, Analysis, and Interpretation in Clinical Trials,* which expands considerably on the statistical concepts presented in this book. Volume 2 will be published in 2012.)

In this case, the *p*-value associated with the test statistic and the Degrees of Freedom is 0.004. Hence, the following numerical result can be stated:

$$t(19) = 3.27, p=0.004$$

This, however, is not the end of the analytical process. These numbers must be interpreted in words in the context of the specific study. Before doing this, however, the concept of *p*-values needs to be considered.

7.3.1 Probability and *p*<0.05

Probability is an important component of Statistics. One commonly used level of probability is the 5% level, a percentage version of odds of one in 20: If the odds of something occurring are one in 20, there is a 5% chance that it will occur. Imagine twenty playing cards lying upside down in a row on a table. You are told that one of them is the 'Ace of Hearts.' You are then asked to select a single card and turn it over. What is the probability that the card you choose will be the Ace of Hearts? There are 20 cards, and each card has the same chance of being chosen as the others. There is only one Ace of Hearts, and so your odds are one in 20, and hence you have a 1 in 20 chance of picking the card. In other words, there is a 5% probability that you will choose the Ace of Hearts.

A probability of 5% can be expressed as $p=0.05$. The statement $p<0.05$ (i.e., a probability that is less than 0.05) means that the odds of something occurring is less than one in 20, i.e., less than 5%. It has become statistical convention that, if the p-value that results from an inferential test is less than 5%, the result is declared to be statistically significant.

The phrase "$p<0.05$" may well be the single most well-known term in drug development. As explained shortly, there must be statistically significant evidence of a drug's efficacy for a regulatory agency to approve it for marketing. However, despite its attained prominence, the value of 0.05 was not ordained: it was conceived by the visionary statistician Sir Ronald Fisher. He could have chosen another value. Had he decided, for example, that odds of one in 25 were more appropriate than odds of one in 20 in this context, the associated p-value would have been 0.04 instead. Whether the value of 0.05 is "right" (whatever right means) is not the issue here. The important point is the acknowledgment that a particular value has been chosen and honored to allow the discipline of Statistics to be beneficially employed: That value is 0.05.

From the present perspective, a statistically significant result is regarded as a probabilistic statement that the result obtained was not a chance occurrence, but was the result of a systematic influence on the data collected from the subjects in the two treatment groups. What systematic influence(s) could have been at work here? This example presents hypothetical data from a randomized, controlled, parallel-groups Phase III clinical trial. The process of randomization was used to ensure that, as far as possible, the subjects in the drug treatment group were similar to those in the placebo treatment group. Hence, the only systematic influence was the treatment administered: the drug was administered to all subjects in the drug treatment group, and the placebo was administered to all subjects in the placebo treatment group. By statistical convention, it is therefore declared that the identified systematic influence, the drug's effect, was responsible for the difference in mean responses between the groups.

7.3.2 Returning to our Example

Once again, here are the hypothetical data from our example (recall that the values represent decreases in MAP from baseline to the end of the treatment period):

- Drug treatment group (N=10): 3, 0, 3, 8, 5, 9, 4, 7, 5, 6.
- Placebo treatment group (N=11): 4, 2, 2, 0, 1, 0, 1, 4, 3, 2, 3.

As seen previously, the result from the statistical analysis is as follows:

$$t(19) = 3.27, p=0.004$$

We can now go further:

1. Since 0.004 is less than 0.05, the test statistic has attained statistical significance at the 0.05 level, and the result can therefore be declared statistically significant. At this point, the test statistic, i.e., 3.27, can be disregarded: it has determined whether or not statistical significance was attained (it was), and the work of the test statistic itself is therefore done.
2. We now know that the mean decreases in MAP in the two treatment groups are statistically significantly different. To find the direction of the difference we need to calculate and compare the two means.
3. The mean MAP decrease for the drug treatment group was 5 mmHg, and the mean MAP decrease for the placebo treatment group was 2 mmHg. Therefore, the drug led to a statistically significantly greater decrease in MAP than did the placebo.

We can now calculate the treatment effect. In the present case, the treatment effect is calculated as the mean decrease in MAP for the drug treatment group minus the mean decrease in MAP for the placebo treatment group. Hence, the treatment effect is 5 mmHg minus

2 mmHg, i.e., 3 mmHg. We can now give a complete answer: The drug lowered blood pressure statistically significantly more than placebo, and its treatment effect was 3 mmHg. This answer provides compelling evidence of statistically significant efficacy.

However—and it is a big "However"— the attainment of statistical significance, while one of the important factors taken into account by regulatory agencies when considering whether or not to grant marketing approval, is not the whole story. Clinical significance must also be considered.

7.4 Clinically Significant Efficacy

As just discussed, the standard by which compelling evidence of statistically significant efficacy is demonstrated is the treatment effect's attainment of the 5% level of statistical significance (i.e., $p<0.05$). However, demonstration of a statistically significant treatment effect is not sufficient. Gardner and Altman (1986) commented that "presenting p-values alone can lead to them being given more merit than they deserve. In particular, there is a tendency to equate statistical significance with medical importance or biological relevance." Statistical significance must not be equated with medical importance or biological relevance. In the clinical arena, the use of confidence intervals is particularly meaningful, and their presentation is an important component of regulatory documentation and clinical communications.

7.4.1 Placement of the Confidence Interval

The treatment effect obtained in our ongoing example is 3 mmHg. It is now appropriate to place a confidence interval around this value, which, as noted earlier, is now referred to as the treatment effect point estimate. In this situation, the two-sided 95% CI is commonly used to determine a range of values that we are 95% confident will cover the true but unknown population treatment effect. The result for these data is:

Limits of the two-sided 95% CI $= 3 \pm X$

In this case, X is calculated to be 1.92 (again, we do not need to present these calculations). Hence we have the following:

Limits of the two-sided 95% CI = 3 ± 1.92 = 1.08 and 4.92

Since there are two decimal places used in the numerical expression of the lower limit and the upper limit, two decimal places have now been used for the treatment effect point estimate, leading to the values being expressed as follows:

95% CI = 3.00 (1.08, 4.92)

The following statement can now be made:
- The data obtained from this single trial are compatible with a treatment effect in the general population as small as 1.08 mmHg and as large as 4.92 mmHg, and our best estimate is 3.00 mmHg.

7.4.2 Interpretation of this Result

Using round numbers for the lower and upper confidence interval limits we can say that, if the drug were to be approved and used in the general population, the data from this single clinical trial suggest that it could lower MAP somewhere in the range of 1 mmHg to 5 mmHg. The question now becomes: Has this result provided compelling evidence of clinically significant efficacy or not?

For any set of data, statistical significance can be evaluated by following the procedural rules of hypothesis testing, a precise formulaic strategy that provides an unequivocal answer that a result either is or is not statistically significant. The process of determining clinical significance, however, is not as straightforward since it is not formulaic and requires skilled clinical judgment. Consider our example involving MAP. In clinical practice, antihypertensive therapy is largely, and successfully, based around certain milestones that represent delineation between normal blood pressure and elevated blood pressure

(JNC, 2004). The practicalities of such large-scale pharmacotherapy are assisted by the development of drugs that have worthwhile efficacy, since all drugs bring with them the potential for side effects: the benefit (efficacy) must outweigh any risk. How, therefore, is 'worthwhile' operationalized? This is a matter of clinical judgment.

Framing this question in another way is helpful: What is the smallest treatment effect that is clinically meaningful, or clinically relevant, and hence can be considered clinically significant? This treatment effect size can be called the clinically relevant difference (CRD). Its determination is a clinical one, not a statistical one. Certainly, this determination will be strongly influenced by existing empirical evidence, but its determination is not simply formulaic. Consider the result from our hypothetical example: If the drug were to be approved and used in the general population, the data from this single clinical trial suggest that it could lower blood pressure somewhere in the range of 1 mmHg to 5 mmHg in the general population of hypertensives. Looking at the top end of this range, this question can be asked: Is it clinically relevant, i.e., clinically significant, to decrease blood pressure by 5 mmHg? The answer may be yes. (Note: The author is not a clinician, and my comments concerning these hypothetical data should be judged in that light.) At the other end of the range of values, the same question can be asked for a decrease in blood pressure of 1 mmHg. Even though theoretically any decrease is to be welcomed, from a practical pharmacotherapy perspective, a drug that may lower MAP by 1 mmHg may not be considered a good candidate for marketing approval since there are likely to be other drugs already on the market that lower it to a greater degree. Hence, the answer to the question "Is a decrease of 1 mmHg clinically significant?" may be no. Therefore, it is possible that a decision would be reached that the data provided by this trial do not provide compelling evidence of clinically significant efficacy, even though they do provide compelling evidence of statistically significant efficacy.

While this may initially sound like a contradiction, it actually provides a good example of the difference between statistical significance and clinical significance. Think of it in these terms. Statistical significance addresses the reliability of the treatment effect: we have compelling evidence that the drug will lower MAP. In contrast, clinical significance addresses the magnitude of the treatment effect. Putting these together, the data from this single trial provide compelling evidence that the drug will lower MAP in the general population of hypertensives, but it is possible that it will reliably lower MAP by only 1 mmHg.

7.5 Emphasizing an Earlier Point

A point made earlier is worth repeating here. The ultimate purpose of the results from a clinical trial is not to tell us precisely what happened in that trial, but to gain insight into likely drug responses in patients who would be prescribed the drug should it be approved for marketing. This is a fundamental concept in assessments of both safety and efficacy. Appropriate analyses of the data from a given trial, i.e., from a given set of subjects who participated in the trial, are used to infer what is likely to be the case for patients in the future.

CHAPTER 8

Integrative Discussion

8.1 Introduction

MAJOR THEMES COVERED by previous chapters include:

- Ethical considerations are of central importance.
- Due attention must be paid to study design, methodological rigor, operational execution, and statistical analysis and interpretation.
- A new drug's safety and efficacy must be thoroughly investigated during its preapproval clinical development program. Safety information is collected in every trial conducted.
- Definitive efficacy assessment comes from the final trials performed before applying for marketing permission, i.e., the Phase III trials that are the focus of this book.
- A drug must demonstrate statistically significant and clinically significant efficacy. Statistical significance is captured by the value of $p<0.05$, while clinical significance is assessed by employing confidence intervals.

8.2 Ethical Considerations

Ethical considerations are pervasive throughout clinical trials. The need for ethical treatment of all subjects who are willing to participate in clinical research is paramount. Also, since it is unethical to include subjects in a study where poor design and/or poor methodology and operational execution leads to less-than-optimum quality data and therefore less-than-optimum answers to the study's research question, everyone involved in clinical research has the responsibility to act in an ethical manner. Ethics are not simply something for 'ethicists or someone else' to worry about. Ethical considerations occur in multiple contexts in clinical trials contexts, including:

- Subject recruitment and retention, including providing informed consent and allowing subjects to withdraw from the trial at any time they wish to.
- When a trial is completed, authors of regulatory documents and manuscripts submitted to peer-reviewed journals for publication have an ethical responsibility to report information accurately since these directly impact patient care.

A quote from Derenzo and Moss (2007) that captures these sentiments very well was presented in Section 1.1, right at the start of the book. It is worth repeating here:

> Each study component has an ethical aspect. The ethical aspects of a clinical trial cannot be separated from the scientific objectives. Segregation of ethical issues from the full range of study design components demonstrates a flaw in understanding the fundamental nature of research involving human subjects. Compartmentalization of ethical issues is inconsistent with a well-run trial. Ethical and scientific considerations are intertwined (p. 4).

8.3 Design, Methodology, Operations, and Analysis

Design, methodology, operational execution, and analysis and interpretation are of great importance in all clinical trials. Early-phase clinical studies involve relatively small numbers of subjects. However, this does not mean that design, methodology, execution, and analysis are any less critical than for later-phase studies involving considerably larger numbers of subjects. Machin and Campbell (2005) noted that these early-phase clinical studies provide key information for designing Phase III trials, and that it is therefore "essential that they are carefully designed, painstakingly conducted, and meticulously reported in full."

8.3.1 A More Expansive Definition of Statistics

The discipline of Statistics was briefly discussed in Section 1.3. At this point, a comprehensive definition of Statistics in the realm of clinical trials and drug development can be provided. Statistics can be thought of as an integrated discipline that is important in all of the following activities (Turner, 2010):

- Identifying a research question that needs to be answered.
- Deciding upon the design of the study, the methodology that will be employed, and the numerical information (data) that will be collected.
- Presenting the design, methodology, and data to be collected in a study protocol. This study protocol specifies the manner of data collection, and addresses all methodological considerations necessary to ensure the collection of optimum quality data for subsequent statistical analysis.
- Identifying the statistical techniques that will be used to describe and analyze the data in the protocol and/or an associated statistical analysis plan, which should be written in conjunction with the study protocol.
- Describing and analyzing the data. This includes analyzing the variation in the data to see if there is compelling evidence that the drug is safe and effective. This process includes evaluation of the statistical significance of the results obtained and, importantly, their clinical significance.
- Presenting the results of a clinical study to a regulatory agency in a clinical study report and presenting the results to the clinical community in journal publications.

Upon first reading it, this definition of Statistics may seem rather expansive, and indeed it is. However, statistical awareness is essential throughout the entire drug development process, from designing a study to answer a research question right through to presenting the study results to regulatory agencies and the clinical community, and therefore an expansive definition is appropriate.

8.3.2 Numerical Representations of Biological Information

The data acquired in a clinical trial are not simply numbers: They are numerical representations of biologically and clinically important information. The number 9 is meaningful by itself (it is an integer between 8 and 10). However, in a clinical database, the digit 9 may represent many things, e.g., a decrease of 9 mmHg seen in a subject's MAP following the administration of an investigational antihypertensive drug for several weeks, or an increase in HDLc following treatment with a drug intended to raise HDLc levels.

8.3.3 Thoughts on *p*-Values

Demonstration of statistically significant efficacy in Phase III trials (i.e., $p < 0.05$) is important. However, demonstration of clinical significance is more important. Piantadosi (2005) commented on this issue as follows:

> Not even a brief discussion of estimation and analysis methods for clinical trials would be complete without an appropriate de-emphasis of *p*-values as the proper currency for conveying treatment effects. There are many circumstances in which *p*-values are useful, particularly for hypothesis tests specified *a priori*. However, they have properties that make them poor summaries of clinical effects…In particular, they do not convey the magnitude of a clinical effect. The size of the *p*-value is a consequence of two things: the magnitude of the estimated treatment difference and its estimated variability (which is itself a consequence of sample size). Thus the *p*-value partially reflects the size of the experiment, which has no biological importance. The *p*-value also hides the size of the treatment, which does have major biological importance (p. 432).

8.4 Confidence Intervals and Clinical Significance

Confidence intervals are extremely informative since, unlike *p*-values, they focus on the magnitude of estimated treatment effect and therefore facilitate consideration of its clinical significance. As Fletcher and Fletcher (2005) observed, confidence intervals "put the emphasis where it belongs, on the size of the [treatment] effect." The width of a confidence interval around an experimentally determined treatment effect point estimate, and hence the range of plausible values for the true but unknown population treatment effect, provides vital information about the clinical significance of the treatment.

8.5 Benefit-risk Estimation

As we have seen, the FDA's Sentinel Initiative (FDA, 2008) provided a useful definition of drug safety in terms of benefit-risk estimation:

> Although marketed medical products are required by federal law to be safe for their intended use, **safety does not mean zero risk**. A safe product is one that has acceptable risks, given the magnitude of benefit expected in a specific population and within the context of alternatives available.

Benefit-risk decisions are made by regulatory agencies whenever approving (or not) a drug for marketing, and when considering removing an approved drug from the market or otherwise restricting its use. Physicians and their patients also make benefit-risk decisions when deciding whether or not a patient should receive a drug.

8.6 Concluding Comments

This book has highlighted the roles of study design, experimental methodology, operational execution, and statistical analysis and interpretation in clinical trials. All of the activities discussed are vital in developing biopharmaceutical drugs that will improve patients' health and well-being. As noted at the start of Chapter 1, drug development is a noble pursuit and it is a privilege to be a part of this process.

If you work in this field, might be interested in doing so in the future, or have read this book because of your interest in clinical medicine, I hope it has helped you to have a better understanding of the clinical trial process and the importance of everyone's contribution.

References

Brown Stafford P, 2011, Moving from Managing Data to Managing Information. Presentation at the 2011 Annual Meeting of the Drug Information Association, June 21st, Chicago, USA.

Cabell C, 2009, Patient recruitment: Are we looking in the right place? *International Pharmaceutical Industry*, Summer issue, 38-41.

Caveney E, Turner JR, 2010, Regulatory landscapes for future anti-diabetic drug development (Part I): FDA guidance on assessment of cardiovascular risks. *Journal for Clinical Studies*, January issue, 34-36.

Chow S-C, Chang, M, 2007, *Adaptive Design Methods in Clinical Trials: Concepts and Methodologies.* CRC/Taylor Francis.

Derenzo E, Moss J, 2006, *Writing Clinical Research Protocols: Ethical Considerations.* Elsevier.

FDA, 2008, The Sentinel Initiative: National Strategy for Monitoring Medical Product Safety.

Fletcher RH, Fletcher SW, 2005, *Clinical Epidemiology*, 4th Edition. Lippincott Williams & Wilkins.

Gardner MJ, Altman DG, 1986, Estimation rather than hypothesis testing: Confidence intervals rather than p-values. In Gardner MJ, Altman DG (Eds), *Statistics with Confidence.* British Medical Association.

Gough J, Hamrell M, 2010, Standard Operating Procedures (SOPs): How companies can determine which documents they must put in place. *Drug Information Journal*, 44:49-54.

Institute of Medicine of the National Academies, 2007, *The Future of Drug Safety: Promoting and Protecting the Health of the Public.* National Academies Press. (Report released September 2006, published in book form in 2007)

Jaishankar R, 2009, Patient recruitment and retention in clinical trials. *International Pharmaceutical Industry*, Spring issue, 26-28.

JNC, 2004, The Seventh Report of the Joint National Committee on Prevention, Detection, Evaluation, and Treatment of High Blood Pressure (JNC 7). [Note: The eighth report in this series, JNC 8, is expected in Spring 2012.]

Machin D, Campbell MJ, 2005, *Design of Studies for Medical Research.* Wiley.

Nada A, Somberg J, 2007, First-in-man (FIM) clinical trials post-TeGenero: A review of the impact of the TeGenero trial on the design, conduct, and ethics of FIM trials. *American Journal of Therapeutics*, 14:594-604.

Piantadosi S, 2005, *Clinical Trials: A Methodologic Perspective*, 2nd Edition. Wiley.

Rosenberg M, 2010, *The Agile Approach to Clinical Research: Optimizing Efficiency in Drug Development.* Wiley.

Salvi V, Panicker GK, Karnad DR, Kothari S, 2010, Update on the evaluation of a new drug for effects on cardiac repolarization in humans: Issues in early drug development. *British Journal of Pharmacology*, 159:34-48.

Satin LZ, Durham TA, Turner JR, 2011, Assessing a drug's proarrhythmic liability: An overview of computer simulation modeling, nonclinical assays, and the Thorough QT/QTc Study. *Drug Information Journal*, 45:357-375.

Spilker B, 2009, *Guide to Drug Development: A Comprehensive Review and Assessment.* Wolters Kluwer/Lippincott Williams & Wilkins.

Turner JR, *New Drug Development: An Introduction to Clinical Trials*, 2nd Edition. New York: Springer.

Turner JR, Caveney S, 2010, Regulatory landscapes for future antidiabetic drug development (Part II): EMA guidance on assessment of cardiovascular risks, *Journal for Clinical Studies*, March issue, 38-40.

Index

About the Author

J. RICK TURNER, PhD, is an experimental research scientist and clinical trialist, and currently Senior Scientific Director, Integrated Cardiovascular Safety, Quintiles. With his colleagues, he provides Sponsors with consultation, strategic and regulatory insights, and operational support during cardiac safety assessments throughout clinical development programs. He is particularly interested in the development of drugs for Type 2 Diabetes Mellitus and obesity.

Dr Turner is also a Senior Fellow at the Center for Medicine in the Public Interest (New York) and Editor-in-Chief of the DIA's peer-reviewed *Drug Information Journal*. He has published 12 previous books, 65 peer-reviewed papers, and many articles in professional journals. His books include:

- Turner JR, 2011, *Key Statistical Concepts in Clinical Trials for Pharma*. New York: Springer.
- Turner JR, 2010, *New Drug Development: An Introduction to Clinical Trials*, 2nd Edition. New York: Springer.
- Turner JR, Durham TA, 2009, *Integrated Cardiac Safety*: *Assessment Methodologies for Noncardiac Drugs in Discovery, Development, and Postmarketing Surveillance*. Hoboken, NJ: John Wiley & Sons.
- Durham TA, Turner JR, 2008, *Introduction to Statistics in Pharmaceutical Clinical Trials*. London: Pharmaceutical Press.

A Concise Guide to Clinical Trials is a publication of Turner Medical Communications LLC, where Dr Turner is President and Chief Scientific Officer.

Made in the USA
Middletown, DE
10 September 2015